KU-050-673

Sport, Exercise and Environmental Physiology

Thomas Reilly BA DipPE MSc PhD DSc DHC FIBiol FErgS

*Director, Research Institute for Sport and Exercise Sciences,
Liverpool John Moores University, Liverpool, UK*

Jim Waterhouse BA(Oxon) DPhil(Oxon)

*Senior Lecturer, Research Institute for Sport and Exercise Sciences,
Liverpool John Moores University, Liverpool, UK*

Foreword by

Richard Budgett OBE

Director of Medical Services, British Olympic Association

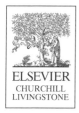

ELSEVIER
CHURCHILL
LIVINGSTONE

EDINBURGH LONDON NEW YORK OXFORD PHILADELPHIA ST LOUIS SYDNEY TORONTO 2005

ELSEVIER
CHURCHILL
LIVINGSTONE

First published 2005

ISBN 0 443 07358 9

British Library Cataloguing in Publication Data
A catalogue record for this book is available from the British Library

Library of Congress Cataloging in Publication Data
A catalog record for this book is available from the Library of Congress

Notice
Knowledge and best practice in this field are constantly changing. As new research and experience broaden our knowledge, changes in practice, treatment and drug therapy may become necessary or appropriate. Readers are advised to check the most current information provided (i) on procedures featured or (ii) by the manufacturer of each product to be administered, to verify the recommended dose or formula, the method and duration of administration, and contraindications. It is the responsibility of the practitioner, relying on their own experience and knowledge of the patient, to make diagnoses, to determine dosages and the best treatment for each individual patient, and to take all appropriate safety precautions. To the fullest extent of the law, neither the publisher nor the authors assume any liability for any injury and/or damage.

The
publisher's
policy is to use
**paper manufactured
from sustainable forests**

Printed in China

613.
71
REI

Contents

Foreword   *vii*

Preface   *ix*

Chapter 1
Exercise and the environment – an ergonomics approach   **1**

Chapter 2
Exercise and the heat   **13**

Chapter 3
Exercise and the cold   **33**

Chapter 4
Altitude stress and hypoxia   **51**

Chapter 5
Underwater sports   **73**

Chapter 6
The stress of travel   **89**

Chapter 7
The effects of space flight   **117**

Chapter 8
Air quality   **145**

Chapter 9
Noise   **165**

Chapter 10
Living and exercising in hostile environments   **181**

Index   193

Foreword

This book is important to all those concerned with health, safety and performance in any environment. As a sports physician, I recognise the importance of environment. The two authors of this book are leaders in their fields, and the book contains cutting-edge research presented in a clear, readable format. The very best information is backed by evidence and expert advice. A variety of issues concerning the protection of individuals and their potential adaptation to extreme environments are discussed and the best solutions are presented. The book contains a wealth of fascinating background information and useful, practical advice, particularly on the stresses of travel, including 'jet lag'.

All those working with athletes, from recreational to elite, will appreciate this book. It is well referenced and can be read through from beginning to end, or used as a reference text.

In preparing for an Olympic Games, I will use the relevant chapters, confident that they provide the latest and most accurate information on how best to tackle problems associated with heat or cold, altitude or air quality, the stress of travel and even noise pollution. Along with the other Olympic support staff, I can then take steps to optimise the protection of the team through acclimatisation, the use of appropriate equipment and carefully planned training sessions.

Dr Richard Budgett OBE
Director of Medical Services,
British Olympic Association

Preface

This book was written to provide a broad view of the relationships existing between humans and the environment they inhabit, and sometimes create. These relationships have become increasingly complex as more and more people test their capabilities not only on hostile terrain but also under water, in space and in extreme conditions.

The focus is on environmental stresses and how people adapt or learn to cope with them. Whilst the main scientific discipline of the authors is physiology, an ergonomics stance is taken throughout. The challenges confronting individuals in difficult situations are not just described: solutions are considered and recommendations made.

The content is more comprehensive than previous texts concerned with the environment and the particular environmental stresses imposed on humans. The material is organised so that the overall concepts of ergonomics are adopted in the first chapter. Temperature extremes embrace hot and cold conditions, and these are included in Chapters 2 and 3. Pressure is then addressed, in the context of altitude (Chapter 4) and underwater environments (Chapter 5). Travel, space, air quality and noise are then treated separately before the harmony between humans and the environments in which they dwell is discussed in the final chapter.

The book should be of interest to a wide range of readers. Within the sports sciences, where environmental physiology is a component of the syllabus, readers might be undergraduates, Masters level students or research workers. The material will also be of relevance to practitioners such as coaches, physiotherapists or sports physicians. It is anticipated that the book will also be appropriate for students in the human sciences, including human factors specialists and ergonomists.

The book is based on experimental and empirical evidence and referenced appropriately. The references allow the reader to search out original sources of evidence and on occasion the reader is directed towards important reviews and textbooks. The focus on the environment and human integration within it provides a unique pedagogical resource for those communities at which the book is targeted.

Thomas Reilly
Jim Waterhouse

Liverpool, 2005

Chapter 1

Exercise and the environment: An ergonomics approach

CHAPTER CONTENTS

Background 1
Fitting the task to the person 2
Human factors criteria 4
The health and safety perspective 5

Standardization of the environment 7
The human–machine interface 8
Overview 10

BACKGROUND

One of the axioms of human activity is that the individual is in harmony with the environment. The environmental context may range from the comparative ease of urban and rural settings to the much more challenging one of the wilderness. The advent of technology has prompted humans to experience and challenge extremes of environmental stresses not naturally accessible to them. Not only are the seas and mountains open to human endeavours, but so too are the depths of underwater exploration and the uncertainties of space travel.

Such adventures expose the human body to extremes of physical and physiological stress. The paradox is that the human spirit continually seeks to conquer new heights, traverse untrammelled territories and achieve feats hitherto unattempted. The unhelpful answer to the question of why people climb a high mountain is 'because it is there'. Even so, it is the same spirit, which is indissolubly linked with being human, that enabled our remote ancestors to tame fire and make metals, our more recent ones to sail to new continents and enables our contemporaries to make plans to visit Mars.

Environmental stresses induce physiological responses to enable the individual to cope. The complex way in which humans interact with their work, leisure and domestic environments has become a serious subject of study. The science of ergonomics (also known as 'human factors') provides a framework for analyzing the relationship between the individual, the activity or task in hand, and the environment in which the activity takes place. The focus is primarily on the individual and how he or she harmonizes with the activity and the prevailing environment. Whilst there is often a need to protect the individual against the environment, the focus in this chapter is on a total integration between the human and the environment.

FITTING THE TASK TO THE PERSON

A fundamental principle of ergonomics is that human characteristics are taken into account when designing the work environment, the equipment to be used and the task to be done. In practice, tasks often have to be redesigned in order for individuals to cope. The designer or planner has to take into account the range of human characteristics (e.g. anthropometry) and capabilities (e.g. maximal power output, reaction time, range of movement, working posture and so on). The principle of 'fitting the task to the human' has been a feature of classical ergonomics. If the task is not fitted to the individual, performance is likely to be below optimum and the resultant strain on the human may cause breakdown or injury.

A feature of competitive sport is that individuals are pushed regularly to their limits. This degree of strain is likely to generate errors and to set in motion a sequence of events that may lead to accidents. Some of these accidents will result in injury. In some environmental circumstances errors in performance (or in decision-making) can be catastrophic for the individual concerned, for example in rock-climbing, hang-gliding or deep-sea diving. In sport, the individual may be protected to some extent by the design of appropriate clothing. In some cases the employment of protective equipment may alter the way games are played, and not always for the better (in American football, for example, the helmet was originally designed to protect the player's head but began to be used as a means of attacking an opponent headfirst). Such safety considerations supplement comfort and fit as criteria in the design of sports footwear, sports clothing and protective equipment to be used in different environmental conditions.

In contemporary society, humans have become processors of information, replacing their traditional function of energy processing. There has been an increasing focus on the use of computers and innovative communication technologies, and on human-computer interaction. The design of 'virtual reality' environments can engage individuals totally, albeit sometimes in a physically passive manner. Computers also have widespread usage within the sports world. Current examples include computer simulations for analyzing sports equipment design, for on-line booking of sports facilities, for analysis of patterns of play in games, for monitoring sailing expeditions and modelling likely climatic conditions. These analytical facilities provide feedback on the myriad of subtle ways in which performance can be improved, competitors' weaknesses exposed, and how performance may break down in certain environmental circumstances. Other examples include the visual representation of hostile conditions to be used by participants, so that mental preparation for the forthcoming event becomes realistic.

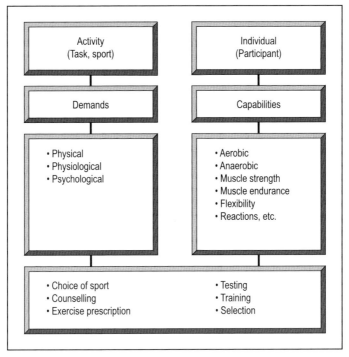

Figure 1.1 An ergonomics model of sports participation. After Reilly T. Sports ergonomics: an introduction[2]

Computer games offer a major recreational facility for young people. Participation is attractive and it is feared that these games distract boys and girls from outdoor pursuits at a time when health-promoting lifestyles should be inculcated. The design of digital interactive computer games utilizes increasingly sophisticated software to engage participants. In some cases the sports competitive environment is modelled very realistically. Participation in 'virtual reality' becomes a substitute for active engagement. The consequences of long-term inactivity are morbidities such as cardiovascular disease, obesity, diabetes and other disorders. Adventurous exercise in wilderness, and exhilarating exploratory activities, provide attractive contrasts to this sedentary lifestyle.

The foundations of ergonomics were laid during the 1940s when the war effort in munitions factories required individual workers to stay on duty for long hours. Despite the huge motivation to do so, productivity was not necessarily improved by working overtime. The notion of fatigue, both physiological and mental, was recognized. Environmental conditions in the munitions factories, notably temperature and light, were not conducive to optimal performance. Individuals monitoring visual displays and looking for occasional signals against a background of noise were prone to loss of concentration and to miss signals. It was acknowledged that humans had a limited capacity and a fundamental swing in thought was that the tasks, the machinery and the work environment should be re-designed to fit human capabilities.

The principles of the classical ergonomics approach were captured in Grandjean's[1] text entitled 'Fitting the Task to the Man'. The classical approach views the selection of individuals and the design of activities and work environments as highly important (see Figure 1.1). The existence of limits helps to emphasize that there is a ceiling to human capabilities, that is reflected in physiological, physical or psychological characteristics. These functions may be overloaded when environmental stresses are encountered. In such cases a compromise must be reached to reduce the load on the individual, or to delegate aspects of the task to mechanical means and to non-human sources of power.

This approach contrasts with many of the principles within competitive sport, where there is a strong dependence on training and pushing back the boundaries of human capabilities. Its parallel in recreational activities is the search to explore ever more challenging and extreme environments.

HUMAN FACTORS CRITERIA

Whilst sports engineers may emphasize the design of clothing, equipment and machines, the human factor must not be forgotten. The matching of task demands and human capabilities is an overriding feature of ergonomics. If the demands are excessive, the result constitutes stress for the individual which will be recorded as physiological strain. This notion applies equally whether the human is processing energy or processing information, whether in the comparative comfort of a factory, out on the sports field, or climbing a mountain.

A principle of ergonomics is that stress should be reduced to keep the operator within a 'comfort zone'. However, some degree of stimulation is essential to keep the individual sufficiently alert so that cognitive function and mental concentration are maintained. A further concept is that the task is accomplished with the greatest efficiency possible. Efficiency refers to the work done as a percentage of the energy expended. This concept of energy-sparing is especially important to individuals exposed to hostile environments for sustained periods. Carrying extra energy reserves in itself can increase the daily outlay of energy.

Probably the most important principle of ergonomics is that of safety (see Table 1.1). It may in fact override all other considerations for legal reasons and professional accountability. Competitive sport carries some degree of injury risk which varies according to the sport, the level of the competition and the prevailing environment. In many outdoor activities, legal responsibility may constrain the behaviour and freedom of movement allowed to participants. In extreme cases, the individual may be confronted with unforeseen ethical dilemmas. For example, to what extent does a struggling climber on the high mountain risk his or her own safety by stopping to help a dying colleague?

Table 1.1 The distinction between ergonomics criteria and engineering criteria

Ergonomics criteria	Engineering criteria
Comfort	Increased output
Stress reduction	Lowered maintenance costs
Increased efficiency	Training requirements
Reduced risk	Ease of operation

THE HEALTH AND SAFETY PERSPECTIVE

The design and layout of the workplace and the competitive sports environment are subject to statutory regulations. The fundamental principle is that the health and safety of the individual are paramount. Therefore all reasonable steps must be taken in order to ensure that risks are minimized.

In the United Kingdom, the Health and Safety at Work Act of 1974 had far-reaching implications which extended into the domain of exercise. The law had many ramifications in sports environments and training facilities, but one serves as an example. No longer could owners of fitness training gymnasia allow customers to exercise unsupervised. This law immediately altered practices in weight training, especially where loose weights were being lifted. Emphasis was placed on safe procedures and codes of operation. Furthermore, attention was directed to layout of the training equipment for ease of use. Later the regulatory framework was extended to require formal risk assessment, placing further emphasis on safety procedures and modifying existing environmental conditions where risks were identified.

Sports scientists must now consider in detail the risks entailed in any experimental procedures. They are also obliged to gain the approval of their local Human Ethics Committee prior to commencing research projects. This applies to studies of environmental physiology, not only those conducted in laboratory chambers in which environmental conditions are varied systematically but also to field studies where conditions may be much less predictable.

A classical model of workspace design is illustrated in Figure 1.2. At the centre are the human and the interface with the task or activity. Environmental factors impinge on the interface, particularly in the operation of machines, equipment or computers. Specific environmental variables can be engineered so that the comfort and efficiency of the individual are facilitated rather than compromised. Factors addressed may include air movement, lighting, noise, vibration and air quality.

The human can often be seen to be the 'weakest link'. Just as human capabilities may be extended by diet and appropriate training, human tolerance levels may also be enhanced. Acclimatization procedures help athletes to perform better in hot conditions and at altitude. The degree of enhancement is itself limited so that eventually a ceiling is reached.

Protective equipment enables individuals to survive in extremely hostile environments, or to extend predicted survival times. Use of supplementary oxygen enabled a generation of climbers to reach the summits of the

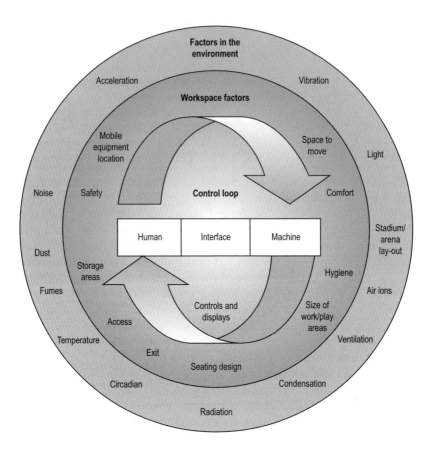

Figure 1.2 Schematic work station analysis map for engineering the total work environment

Himalayan peaks. Cold-protective clothing provides safety for outdoor pursuits whilst crash helmets cushion impacts in machine sports. Whereas the use of protective equipment may be associated with the disadvantage that it encourages the vehicle driver to travel at extreme speed, the abandonment of such protection would be unacceptable.

Researchers into safety may focus on detailed analysis of events that lead to accidents, whatever the environment, examining the possibilities of machine or equipment failure, or human error. An alternative is to focus on 'critical incidents', in which an accident almost took place. Only some errors lead to accidents and only some of these lead to injury (Figure 1.3). Incidents occur far more frequently than accidents or injuries, and so more data are available for analysis. The approach is useful in highlighting predisposing risk factors and also in injury prevention where activities are potentially hazardous. It is also useful in establishing whether critical incidents are attributable to human error or to environmental changes. Such insights provide important information for future endeavours.

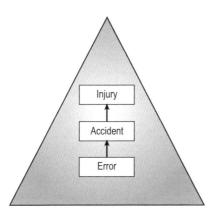

Figure 1.3 The 'critical incident' chain of events

STANDARDIZATION OF THE ENVIRONMENT

Regulations and standards have become an integral part of the application of ergonomics and physiology. There has been an impressive amount of activity devoted to the production of international ergonomics standards since the establishment of the International Organisation for Standardisation (ISO) in 1947. This body co-ordinates the production of internationally accepted standards and over one hundred countries are involved in the process. The standards are revised on a regular basis; their history and development have been reviewed by Parsons et al.[4] Environmental factors subject to standards include the thermal environment, ventilation, acoustics, vibration and so on. Whilst each of these factors can be explored in detail, the appropriate environmental light level is considered here, to illustrate the relevance of standards.

Vision is the mostly widely used human sensory modality in perception of the environment and is a key function in occupational work and sport. There are statutory requirements for lighting, based on safety criteria, which are subject to legislation, at least throughout the European Union. Yet there is also non-statutory guidance on lighting widely available, including aesthetic as well as engineering aspects.

Light refers to radiant energy that can excite the retina and produce a visual sensation. It can be measured in terms of its intensity, flux, illuminance and luminance. Standards for suitable indoor lighting are set as intensities and measured in lux. About 2000 lux with good contrast is required for precision work, 1000 lux for general office work and 100 lux for non-work areas.[5]

The importance of matching light characteristics for sports performance is recognized by various national governing bodies. The regulations for badminton indicate the artificial lighting support needed for competitive matches in indoor halls. Failing light is a common cause of delaying or abandoning cricket matches, as it is in lawn tennis competitions towards the end of the day. Sports such as soccer are now played at elite level largely under floodlit conditions. Most often the lights are turned on at half-time in afternoon matches in the English winter and night-time matches are commonplace.

Visual display units (VDUs) are now widespread in almost all workplaces. Eye discomfort and musculoskeletal illness are the main problems reported by VDU operators. Technical developments have meant that screens now give less flicker than before, more optical contrast and multi-colour flexibility. It has been possible to increase lighting levels in accordance with recommendations for technical office work. Office lighting levels recommended depend on the age profile of the workforce and are in the range 500-10000 lux.[6] The Annex to the Display Screen Directive specifies that the lighting conditions should be satisfactory, with glare avoided by the layout and range of the light fittings, and that adjustable secondary lighting should be available as required.

The alternation of light and darkness has a fundamental effect on human physiology in that it regulates the circadian rhythm in sleep-wakefulness. Darkness triggers the secretion of melatonin from the pineal gland and promotes drowsiness, preparing the body for sleep. The advent of artificial light – both inside and outside – has altered the nocturnal environment, especially in urban areas. Here too, design standards dictate the engineered environment, not only artificial lighting but also noise and pollution thresholds. Social acceptability, as well as safety, is an important criterion.

THE HUMAN–MACHINE INTERFACE

Human physiological capabilities have been enhanced considerably by the availability of technology. Appropriately powered machines have enabled humans to conquer and to understand many of nature's great forces. Their design has extended the range of leisure and adventure activities, from hot-air ballooning to powerboat racing, from scuba diving in ocean waters to skiing on mountain slopes.

The interface between the human and the machine has long been a concern of the ergonomist. The skill of the designer is to optimise the characteristics of each in the production of an effective unit. The best features of each can be compared according to the list shown in Table 1.2. The right combination will enhance the human's capabilities to cope with the physiological stresses of the prevailing work environment.

An example of the fit between human and machine is provided by the challenge of human-powered flight – an endeavour that posed a problem for designers and adventurers for centuries. The task required a human operator to produce muscular power output at approximately 300 W whilst at the same time controlling the pitch, roll and yaw of the craft. A high level of energy expenditure was called for, concomitant with the cognitive demands of controlling the machine in three dimensions. The prize was eventually achieved in the late 1970s by a professional cyclist, Brian Allen, who rode the

Table 1.2 Human vs. machine characteristics

The Human Excels In	Machine Excels In
Detection of certain forms of very low energy levels.	Monitoring (both men and machines).
Sensitivity to an extremely wide variety of stimuli.	Performing routine, repetitive, or very precise operations.
Perceiving patterns and making generalisations about them.	Responding very quickly to control signals.
Detecting signals in high noise levels.	Exerting great force, smoothly and with precision.
Ability to store large amounts of information for long periods - and recalling relevant texts at appropriate moments.	Storing and recalling large amounts of information in short-time periods.
Ability to exercise judgement where events cannot be completely defined.	Performing complex and rapid computation with high with high accuracy.
Improvising and adapting flexible procedures.	Sensitivity to stimuli beyond the range of human sensitivity (infrared, radio waves etc.)
Ability to react to unexpected low-probability events.	Doing many different things at one time.
Applying originality in solving problems: i.e. alternate situations.	Deductive processes.
Ability to profit from experience and alter course of action.	Insensitivity to extraneous factors.
Ability to perform fine manipulation, especially where misalignment appears unexpectedly.	Ability to repeat operations very rapidly, continuously, and precisely the same way over a long period of time.
Ability to continue to perform even when overloaded.	Operating in environments which are hostile to man or beyond human tolerance.
Ability to reason inductively.	

Gossamer machines over a figure-of-eight half-mile course, and subsequently across the English Channel.

Even basic sports equipment must be selected according to environmental conditions. Kinoshita and Bates[7] demonstrated that jogging shoes which contain a moderately hard midsole of ethylene vinyl acetate can be appropriate for moderate ambient temperatures but not for cold or hot conditions. At low temperatures, soft shoes provided a suitable level of shock attenuation and better rearfoot control – factors relevant to injury prevention – than did moderately firm shoes. In high ambient temperatures, firmer shoes were needed to give sufficient rearfoot control. Ordinary running shoes with moderate midsole hardness provide inadequate cushioning in cold and inadequate rearfoot control in hot environments.

People often seek thrills in sporting activities, even though there may be risks involved. Great public interest over many years has centred on fun fairs, fairgrounds and adventure leisure parks. Particular attractions have been the 'merry-go-round', 'roller-coaster' and 'big dipper' devices. Indeed many leisure parks entice participation in activities that can be expected to cause acute psychological reactions among individuals. The motivation for taking part in such activities is not immediately apparent, nor is the magnitude of the strain involved. Reilly et al.[8] studied nine women who undertook a 95-second ride on the 'corkscrew' track at Alton Towers Leisure Park, measuring plasma FFA (free fatty acids), glucose, cortisol and catecholamines under resting control, pre-ride and immediately post-ride conditions. Mood factors of anxiety and thrill were scored by means of a self-evaluation questionnaire before and after the ride. Peak acceleration force obtained from film recordings was 3.5 G (3.5 times that due to gravity) while peak heart rates measured by radio telemetry varied among individuals from 150 to 186 beats/min. Changes in heart rate were associated with abrupt alterations in G forces and in body orientation. Physiological variables, while differing between the conditions, were more strongly related to anxiety than to thrill factors. Subjects showed a habituation effect on subsequent exposure to the ride, reflected in lower concentrations of cortisol, adrenaline and noradrenaline than were evident in the blood after the initial ride. The results indicated a fast adaptation to this acute form of stress as the fear and uncertainty associated with experiencing high G forces were eliminated.

There are many other sports where recreation participants seek thrills by defying natural laws. They include sky diving, parachuting and bungee jumping. Participation stimulates the central nervous system and excites neurotransmitters that affect the pleasure centres of the brain. It is a curious quirk of human nature that fear and anxiety are more than compensated for by the excitement and satisfaction of experiencing such activity.

OVERVIEW

There are many ways in which the environment and its variations can be studied. Physiological studies enable us to understand how the individual responds to environmental stresses whilst ergonomics provides an interdisciplinary perspective in which the relationship between the individual athlete or recreational participant and the environment can be understood. Many activities take place in inhospitable surroundings, which often constitute their inherent challenge. There is no escaping the risks associated with activity in hostile environments. A knowledge of the physiological consequences of exposure to such conditions and methods of coping in emergencies is necessary for those responsible for organizing such outdoor events.

In this chapter, the human's weaknesses and vulnerability to environmental stresses have been emphasized. An ergonomics model places human capabilities in context, and considers the ways in which equipment design helps integrate the individual with the immediate environment. In the remainder of this book, various sources of environmental stress are considered in turn. The physiological responses to each of these stresses are dealt with, along with the means of coping with and training for them.

References

1. Grandjean E. Fitting the task to the man. London: Taylor and Francis, 1988
2. Reilly T. Sports ergonomics: an introduction. In: Advances in sport, leisure and ergonomics. Reilly T, Greeves J (eds). London: Routledge, 2002:3-10
3. Reilly T. Sports fitness and sports injuries. London: Faber and Faber, 1981
4. Parsons KC, Shackel B, Metz B. Ergonomics and industrial standards: history, organisational structure and method of development. Appl Ergon 1995; 26:249-258
5. Oborne DJ. Ergonomics at work. Chichester: John Wiley, 1995
6. Aaras A, Horgen G, Byomet H-H et al. Musculoskeletal, usual and psychological stress in VDU operators before and after multidisciplinary ergonomic evaluations. Appl Ergon 1998; 25:335-354
7. Kinoshita H, Bates BT. The effect of environmental temperature on the properties of running shoes. J Appl Biomech 1996; 12:258-268
8. Reilly T, Lees A, MacLaren D et al. Thrill and anxiety in adventure leisure parks. In: Contemporary ergonomics. Oborne DJ (ed). London: Taylor and Francis, 1985:210-214

Chapter 2

Exercise and the heat

CHAPTER CONTENTS

The environment 13
Physiology of thermoregulation 16
Measurement of body temperature
  17
Effects of heat on performance 19
Heat acclimatization 22

Heat injury 25
Age and gender 27
Monitoring environmental temperature
  28
Overview 30

THE ENVIRONMENT

The environmental temperature in which athletes have to compete or train is rarely conducive to optimal performance. Often, the athlete may be endangered in extremes of heat by a risk of hyperthermia. Climatic factors to consider are ambient temperature, humidity, radiant heat, air velocity, cloud cover and precipitation (rain, sleet and so on).

The human body gains or loses heat according to prevailing conditions and can modify heat exchange with the environment by appropriate behaviour such as exercise and choice of clothing (Table 2.1).

The body can be considered as a 'black box' since it absorbs heat well but also radiates heat to the environment. Heat may be gained from terrestrial sources of radiation or from solar radiation; the body may also gain radiant heat reflected from road surfaces, snow or water. Black surfaces absorb radiant heat whereas white surfaces reflect it. For this reason it has been thought that light-coloured clothing would bestow an advantage over dark-coloured material when athletes exercise in the heat without shade from the sun. Dark clothing would be better in the snow and cold, unless the subjects warm up, when this dark clothing will radiate out heat. The colour of Arctic foxes and polar bears is more a matter of camouflage than heat balance.

The transfer of heat by movement of gas or fluid is referred to as convective heat exchange. The movement of air over the skin surface is an important means of cooling the body when competing in hot conditions,

Table 2.1 Mechanisms of heat exchange

Heat Production (Gain)	Heat loss
Convection (C)	Evaporation (E)
Radiation (R)	Convection (C)
Conduction (K)	Radiation (R)
Activity	Conduction (K)
Shivering	
Increased basal metabolism	
Basal metabolism	

$M - S = E \pm C \pm R \pm K$
M = metabolic heat production, S = storage)

since this movement dispels the layer of warm air adjacent to the skin.

Heat may be transferred from the body core to its surface by means of conduction. The exchange of heat through this physical mechanism is also possible when the skin is in direct contact with materials, surfaces or objects. The material of the clothing and the subcutaneous adipose tissue constitute barriers against heat loss by conduction. Films of stationary air or water in immediate contact with clothing, along with the air trapped in the clothing itself, provide barriers to heat exchange between the body and the environment.

Heat is also lost by the process of evaporation, the rate being determined by the vapour pressure gradient across the film of stationary air surrounding the skin and by the thickness of the stationary film. Evaporation becomes the main avenue for losing heat when exercise is undertaken in hot conditions. Evaporative heat loss occurs with breathing, as water from moist mucous membranes in the upper respiratory tract is vaporized. The result is a gradual dehydration as can happen in dry air, especially at altitude or on board aircraft. Evaporative loss from the lungs is in fact dependent on the minute ventilation, the barometric pressure and the dryness of the air. There is also insensible perspiration through the skin and, as the body temperature rises, there is a secretion of sweat onto the skin surface for the purpose of losing heat by evaporation. In this respect the human is more gifted by evolution than the dog, who lacks sweat glands and depends on the panting mechanism to lose heat via the mouth and upper respiratory tract.

When water evaporates from any surface, that surface is cooled. No heat is exchanged when sweat is produced, but the droplets fall from the skin. The body contains up to two million corkscrew-shaped eccrine sweat glands, located in the dermal layer above the subcutaneous tissue and variously distributed throughout the body. The glands are supplied with cholinergic nerve fibres and are stimulated when the core temperature rises. They differ in type from the apocrine glands (located primarily in the axilla, groin, palms of the hand and soles of the feet) which are supplied by noradrenergic fibres and respond to emotional stimuli.

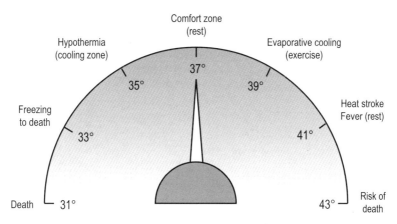

Heat stored = metabolic rate − evaporation ± radiation ± convection ± conduction − work done

Figure 2.1 The zones of body temperature responses

Despite large fluctuations in environmental conditions, core body temperature is normally maintained within a narrow range about a mean of 37°C (see Figure 2.1). The temperature in the periphery of the body is more variable but mean skin temperature is normally about 4°C below core temperature, thus providing a gradient for dissipating heat from the internal organs – heart, viscera and brain. The size of the gradient between the skin and the environment is one of the factors that determines the amount of heat that is lost or gained by the body.

PHYSIOLOGY OF THERMOREGULATION

The body generates heat at rest by its metabolic processes. Heat production may be increased 25-fold during strenuous exercise, around 20% of this contributing to useful work. The remaining 80% is dissipated internally, causing first muscle temperature and then core temperature to rise.

The first main mechanism for losing heat and maintaining thermal balance is by distributing more of the cardiac output through the skin where heat is off-loaded from the 'shell' to the environment. Secondly, sweat is secreted onto the body's surface where it can evaporate. Evaporation is the main means of losing heat during exercise, but the mechanism is obstructed in high relative humidity when the environment is already highly saturated with water vapour. As cardiac output serves both thermoregulation and the transport of oxygen to active muscles, the exercise itself must be reduced to avoid a further rise in core temperature.

A secondary effect of thermoregulation is that the fluid lost in evaporation can result in hypohydration if more body fluid is being lost through sweating than can be restored by fluid intake and its absorption. Thermoregulatory controls override those of body water regulation, as fluid is lost following

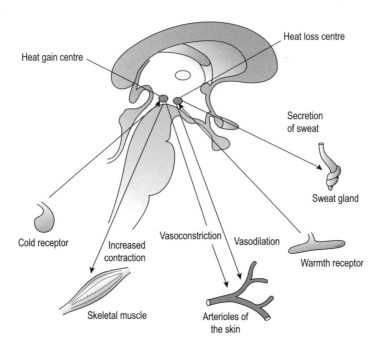

Figure 2.2 Nervous control of temperature regulation

stimulation of the eccrine sweat glands. Dehydration also leads to a deterioration in performance, particularly in events affected by lowered plasma volume. One outcome is a decline in venous return, as a result of which the heart rate rises continuously to maintain blood pressure, a phenomenon known as 'cardiovascular drift'. Therefore progressive loss of fluid compounds the consequences of the rise in body temperature beyond its optimum level.

The temperature of the circulating blood is detected by specialized neurones in the hypothalamus; cells in the anterior portion respond to a temperature rise, cells in the posterior part, to a fall. These areas also receive afferent information from skin receptors about changes in the temperature in the body's immediate environment (see Figure 2.2).

The anterior hypothalamus initiates vasodilation of the skin's circulation when it is necessary to offload heat to the environment. A balance is effected (largely by the hormones renin and angiotensin) whereby vasodilation does not compromise blood pressure. Whilst the sweat glands are activated by sympathetic cholinergic nerve fibres, vasoactive substances from the glands also increase blood flow. Normally the body acts as a heat sink at the beginning of exercise; sweat droplets appear on the skin's surface after about 7 minutes of exercise at 70% of maximal oxygen uptake in temperatures around 20°C.

MEASUREMENT OF BODY TEMPERATURE

Core temperature refers to the thermal state of essential internal organs such as the brain, heart, liver and viscera. It is normally considered that core temperature is regulated about 37°C, but this value varies depending on the site of measurement. The temperature set point also varies during exercise, in fever and according to circadian and circamensal rhythms.

The most commonly used site for measuring core temperature in athletes is the rectum. The measuring probe should be inserted to a depth of 8 cm beyond the external anal sphincter if reliable measures are to be obtained. Care is also needed in ensuring that probes are sterilized and treated with HIV risk in mind. Rectal probes should be washed in warm soapy water and then immersed in a 1:20 concentration of sterilization fluid for at least 30 minutes. On removal from the solution, the probes should be left to dry completely in room air before further use. Skin probes also can be washed and immersed in a 1:40 concentration of sterilization fluid for 10 minutes and then left to dry.

Rectal temperature is not the best measure of core temperature in situations where temperature is changing rapidly. For this reason oesophageal temperature is preferred in some exercise experiments. Measurement entails inserting a probe through the nose and threading it into the oesophagus.

Tympanic temperature is an alternative whereby a sensor is placed adjacent to the tympanic membrane. Caution is necessary as it is easy to damage the membrane and also the ear must be completely insulated to avoid environmental influences. The temperature within the external

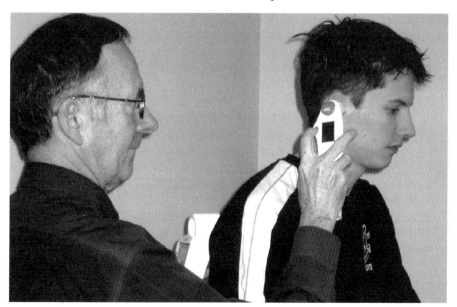

Figure 2.3 The measurement of intra-aural temperature

auditory meatus can also be measured by inserting a probe 1 cm inside the ear canal and insulating the ear. The most common method for measuring intra-aural temperature is with an infra-red device (see Figure 2.3). With this measurement and those of rectal and oesophageal temperatures, it is best to represent data as a change from baseline since a temperature gradient exists between these tissues.

Sublingual or oral temperatures, typically measured with a mercury thermometer, are used in clinical rather than exercise contexts and give values about 0.4°C lower than rectal temperature. Oral temperature is of little use in swimmers, for example, whose mouths are affected by surrounding water and high ventilation rates. Measurement of axilla or groin temperatures in athletic subjects also gives a poor indication of their thermal status, even when the probe is thermally insulated from the environment. A radio-sensitive pill which can be swallowed and then monitored by radio-telemetry has been used in occupational contexts. Difficulties include the necessity for accurate calibration, differences in temperature between the internal organs adjacent to the passage of the pill, the influences of recently digested food on core temperature and the unsavoury task of its retrieval once the pill has traversed the full course of the digestive tract. A more acceptable alternative is to use disposable pills and a data logger worn as a 'bun-bag' by the subject for receiving and recording the signal transmitted. This method has been found to compare favourably with rectal temperature measurement during studies of habitual activity.[1] A further practical option is to measure the temperature of mid-stream urine, which gives a reasonable indication of internal body temperature. However, it is unreliable if urine volumes are small, as is likely to be the case in a warm environment or if sweating has been profuse. It is also inconvenient in conditions of inclement weather, due to the difficulty of obtaining a urine sample in such circumstances.

Skin temperature has conventionally been measured by thermistor and thermocouples. Opto-electronic devices are now also available. The common method is to place thermistors over the surface of the skin and tape over them. From measurements at a number of designated skin sites, a mean skin temperature may be calculated. The formulae[2,3] that require the least number of observations are:

$$MST = 0.5\,T_c + 0.36\,T_1 + 0.14\,T_a$$
$$MST = 0.3\,T_c + 0.3\,T_a + 0.2\,T_t + 0.2\,T_1$$

where MST is mean skin temperature,
T_c is temperature of the chest juxta nipple,
T_1 is leg temperature measured over the lateral side of the calf muscle,
T_a is lower arm temperature,
and T_t is thigh temperature.

Mean body temperature (MBT) may then be calculated by weighting rectal temperature (T_r) and MST in the ratio 4:1. In other words:

$$MBT = 0.8\,T_r + 0.2\,MST.$$

Miniature electronic devices such as the Squirrel data-logger can be used to monitor both core and skin temperatures. The equipment permits the continuous measurement of thermoregulatory responses to environmental conditions so that potentially dangerous rises in heat stress can be identified. Multi-channel data-loggers permit the simultaneous recording of other relevant physiological responses such as heart rate and muscle tension.

Muscle temperature may be recorded by the insertion of a thin needle through the skin into the muscle. This measurement is more suitable for studies in laboratory conditions or in heat chambers although it has been used in field studies, such as at half-time and at the end of football games.

EFFECTS OF HEAT ON PERFORMANCE

Elevation of muscle temperature by 1-2°C facilitates performance and reflects the benefit of a pre-competitive warm-up. An active warm-up by means of light to moderate exercise is more effective than passive warming. A duration of 15-20 minutes seems optimal since sustaining a longer warm-up may contribute to an earlier onset of fatigue in the event that follows. Even at half-time in field games where there is an intermission of 15 minutes, performance at the beginning of the second period is improved if re-warming is commenced half-way through the interval.[4]

A major purpose of warming up prior to performing strenuous exercise is to reduce the risk of muscle injury. The warm-up is most effective in injury prevention when the major muscle groups to be utilized are targeted in the exercise regimen employed.[5] A further benefit is that performance is likely to be enhanced. Metabolic processes within the muscles are speeded up and the rise in blood flow to them means that oxygen is exchanged from the blood to the active tissues at a faster rate.[6] Nerve impulses are transmitted more quickly as temperature increases, which partly accounts for the benefits of warming up for the sprinter as well as for competitors in events which tax the oxygen transport system.

When body temperature rises beyond an optimal value, the level of performance may begin to decline. The ideal environmental temperature for optimal performance will depend on the type of exercise involved, the fitness and heat tolerance of the individual and the combination of environmental variables that prevails. The temperature that is compatible with endurance performance outdoors is much lower than that conducive to thermal comfort for the sedentary person indoors. Whereas the latter is satisfied with a room temperature of 20-21°C, the best performances in marathon races tend to be when ambient temperature is roughly 6°C lower than this value.

Whilst the secretion of sweat helps to avoid overheating, it leads to a gradual loss of body water. This loss of body water leads to increased demands on the circulatory system where thermoregulation is concerned. An athlete exercising in hot conditions may lose up to 2 litres of body water in one hour and higher rates of sweat loss have been reported in marathon runners. Hypohydration leads to progressive impairment of exercise

Table 2.2 Correlations with osmolality (freezing point depression) n = 183[9]

Specific gravity (urinometer)	r = 0.86
Specific gravity (reagent strip)	r = 0.78
Colour (1 - 8 scale chart)	r = 0.63
Conductivity (continuous scale)	r = 0.76

performance, as indicated by both laboratory-based criteria and field measures. The declines are evident in both cognitive and motor components of performance.

Acute thermal dehydration alters the metabolic responses to exercise. England et al.[7] found that blood lactate was increased after a 5% loss of body weight induced passively in a sauna, the elevation in lactate response to exercise being evident at 90, 120 and 150 Watts. Furthermore, the anaerobic threshold (defined as the onset of blood lactate accumulation) occurred at a lower oxygen uptake when the subjects were dehydrated, and the mean time to exhaustion in an incremental test was decreased from 21.5 to 18.0 minutes. It seems that dehydration causes an increased reliance on muscle glycogen as a fuel for exercise.

In field games, where the activity is intermittent and acyclical, the high-intensity bouts of exercise are mainly affected. The distance covered in such efforts declined by about 40% at a temperature of 30°C compared to 20°C.[8] Players have to learn to pace their activity levels to suit prevailing conditions and to replace fluid when breaks in play permit. Whilst the optimal ambient temperature for marathon running is around 14°C for top runners, this value may be too low for those unable to run fast enough to maintain heat balance.

The effect of fluid loss on performance will depend on the degree of hypohydration incurred and the nature of the activity. Effects will be more apparent in sustained activities, where the exercising muscles need to be supplied continuously with oxygen carried in the circulatory system, than in short-term events that depend on anaerobic metabolism. A fluid loss of 2% body mass has been sufficient in most studies to demonstrate a drop in performance. Fluid is lost from all body water pools, including plasma, intramuscular and interstitial fluid.

A water deficit of 1% of body weight leads to a sensation of thirst. This signal is due to a change in cellular osmolality and to dryness in the mucous membrane of the mouth and throat. The feeling of thirst may be satisfied before the fluid lost is fully replaced, indicating that short-term reliance on this mechanism is insufficient. Urine osmolality is probably the best practical physiological marker for monitoring the hydration status of athletes engaged in training in the heat, although urine conductivity is also easily measured and the colour of the urine is a more visible indicator. The correlation of other measures with urine osmolality (Table 2.2) suggests that specific gravity is also an acceptable alternative. The urine becomes more concentrated as the body attempts to retain water by secreting anti-diuretic hormone from the posterior part of the pituitary gland.

Sweat contains electrolytes, urea and lactic acid, the concentrations varying according to the site on the body, whether sweating was actively or passively induced and the fitness level of the individual. There seems to be a large variability between individuals, both in the amount of sweat lost and its sodium concentration. Sweat is hypotonic relative to plasma, reflecting the body's conservation of its sodium content by the secretion of aldosterone. Therefore the main need in fluid replacement when exercising in the heat is for water, both to reduce the rise in body temperature and to restore partially the water lost in sweat. Nevertheless, absorption of the fluid ingested is facilitated if some sodium is included in the drink. The incorporation of energy from sports drinks is relevant in endurance events where there is a likelihood of carbohydrate stores in the muscles and liver running low. In hot conditions it is good practice to start the competition already well hydrated and to take small amounts of fluid on board as occasion allows during the contest. Nevertheless, a quantity of 150 ml every 10-15 minutes is still inadequate to compensate for the losses that can occur, so that in hot conditions a water deficit is inevitable. It is essential that this deficit is made good by replacement of fluid once exercise or training is terminated. Merely calculating the loss of body mass is not enough, since some allowance should be made for the production of urine. As a general guideline it is recommended that an extra 50 ml should be added to the 100 ml implied by a loss of body mass of 100 g.

In sports where there are competitive weight classes, there is a convention of losing weight by dehydrating in order to compete in the lowest possible category. Boxers and wrestlers in particular lose weight before their events to keep within the prescribed limit whilst jockeys also must operate according to the loads outlined for their mounts. The practice is recognized as dangerous, especially if the forthcoming contest is held in hot conditions and severe levels of dehydration have been induced before the formal weigh-in. The use of dehydration as a strategy for making the desired weight has been roundly condemned and in some cases is replaced by a more systematic programme of weight control based on nutritional advice. When a weight loss of 5.2% body weight was incurred over a one-week period by a group of amateur boxers using a combination of food and fluid restriction, performance was found to be reduced.[10] The drop in performance was accompanied by negative moods that included increased anger, fatigue and tension and reduced vigour.

One problem with an aggressive educational programme about fluid replacement is the possibility of overcompensating and incurring hyponatraemia. This term refers to over-dilution of body fluids, causing the sodium (Na) content of the blood to be unduly lowered. It came to notice initially as a problem with South African miners who worked in hot conditions and drank profusely during long work-shifts. In extreme cases,

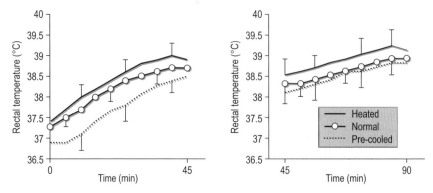

Figure 2.4 The effects of pre-cooling on body temperature during exercise simulating the work-rate of soccer match-play. After Drust B, Cable NT, Reilly T. Investigation of the effects of pre-cooling on the physiological responses to soccer-specific intermittent exercise[13]

over-hydration can induce water toxicity and necessitate hospitalization. The condition has been noted in ultra-marathons and 'ironman triathlons' but presents itself only in avid water drinkers.

The rise in body temperature can be a limiting factor when exercising in the heat, since exhaustion can occur before glycogen stores are depleted. The suggestion is that there is a critical brain temperature that causes central fatigue and acts to protect against heat injury. Cooling the body prior to the start of exercise should increase the time taken to reach this critical temperature. This rationale has led to the adoption of 'pre-cooling' methods immediately before competitive engagements. Hessemer and co-workers[11] showed that reducing oesophageal temperature by 0.5°C and mean skin temperature by 4.5°C before 60 minutes of submaximal exercise helped to improve power output by 6.8%. Olschewski and Bruck[12] reported that a similar reduction in core body temperature caused an extension to cycling time to exhaustion from 18.5 to 20.8 minutes. The effect may be of little benefit to the sprinter who must maintain an elevated muscle temperature to facilitate maximal force production. It may also be lost during games. Drust et al.[13] reported that the effect of pre-cooling prior to a simulation of the work-rate of soccer disappeared after the first 45 minutes (see Figure 2.4).

HEAT ACCLIMATIZATION

The main features of heat acclimatization are an earlier onset of sweating (sweat produced following a smaller rise in body temperature) and a more dilute secretion from the sweat glands (Box 2.1). Loss of sodium in sweat and urine is reduced due to the action of the hormone aldosterone. The heat-acclimatized individual sweats more than an unacclimatized counterpart at a given exercise intensity. There is also a better distribution of blood to the skin for more effective cooling after a period of acclimatization, although such an individual depends more on evaporative sweat loss than on blood flow.

Box 2.1 Characteristics of the acclimatization process

Earlier onset of sweating

Sweat more dilute

Increased sweat rate at same core temperature

Reduced heart rate at a given exercise intensity

Improved pacing of effort

Box 2.2 Pre-acclimatization strategies

(i) The athlete should seek out the hottest time of day to train at home, thereby being exposed to the highest heat load available naturally.

(ii) If the conditions at home are too cool, an environmental chamber may be used for periodic bouts of heat exposure. It is important to exercise rather than rest under such conditions. About 3 hours per week exercising in an environmental chamber are recommended.

(iii) The microclimate next to the skin may be kept hot by wearing heavy sweat suits or windbreakers. This will add to the heat load imposed under cool environmental conditions and induce a degree of adaptation to thermal strain.

(iv) Repeated exposure to a sauna or Turkish bath is only partially effective.

Heat acclimatization occurs relatively quickly and is practically complete within 10-14 days of the initial exposure. Such adaptations enhance the athlete's capability to perform well under heat stress. Ideally, therefore, the athlete or team should be exposed to the climate of the host country for at least 10 days before the event. An alternative is to have an acclimatization period of two weeks or so, well before the event, with subsequent shorter exposures nearer the contest. If these are not practicable, attempts should be made to realize some degree of adaptation to heat before the athlete leaves for the host country. This may be achieved by 'pre-acclimatization' and is a strategy often used by sports teams (see Box 2.2).

On first exposure to a hot climate, athletes should be encouraged to drink copiously to maintain a pale straw-coloured rather than dark urine. They should drink much more fluid than they think they need, since thirst is often a very poor indicator of real need. On arrival in the hot country they should be discouraged strongly from sunbathing as this itself does not help acclimatization except by means of a suntan which eventually protects the skin from damage via solar radiation. Exposure to the sun is not beneficial in the short-term and negative effects of sunburn include discomfort and a decline in performance. Use of a high-factor sunscreen is recommended for those likely to be exposed to sunburn.

Initially, training should be undertaken in the cooler parts of the day for an adequate workload to be achieved, and adequate fluid must be taken regularly. Arrangements should be made to sleep in an air-conditioned environment but adequate acclimatization requires part of the rest of the day to be spent exposed to the ambient temperature. Although sweating increases with acclimatization, the ingestion of salt tablets is not necessary, provided adequate amounts of salt are taken with normal food.

In the acclimatization period the athlete should regularly monitor body weight and try to compensate for weight loss with adequate fluid intake. Alcohol is inappropriate for rehydration purposes since it is a diuretic and increases urine output. Athletes can check that the volume of urine is as large as usual and that its colour is normal. Groups using warm-weather training camps should have urine osmolality (or conductance) monitored regularly to gauge hydration status.

The thermal strain on the individual depends on the relative exercise intensity ($\%\dot{V}O_{2\ max}$) rather than the absolute workload. The higher the maximal aerobic power ($\dot{V}O_{2\ max}$) and cardiac output, the lower the thermal strain on the athlete. Well-trained individuals have a highly developed cardiovascular system to cope with the dual roles of thermoregulation and oxygen delivery. Highly trained individuals also acclimatize more quickly than those who are unfit. Training improves exercise tolerance in the heat but does not eliminate the necessity of heat acclimatization.

Athletes may use warm-weather training camps in order to acclimatize in preparing themselves for major tournaments or championships to be held in hot conditions. These camps would typically be in a location with similar climatic conditions to those anticipated at the competitive venue. For the three years prior to the 1996 Olympic Games, the British Olympic Association used as its base facilities in Tallahassee, Florida, which has the same climate as Atlanta. The England football team used a short sojourn in Dubai to aid acclimatization *en route* to the World Cup in Japan in 2002. Sometimes the climatic conditions do not match in both dry bulb temperature and relative humidity, in which case a combination index such as corrected effective temperature or the WBGT (wet bulb, globe temperature) is used to compare the suitability of the total thermal burden.

Where it is not possible to travel to a hot country to acclimatize, some physiological adjustments may be obtained at home. Use of extra 'sweat clothing' or windbreakers can raise body temperature more than normal and stimulate the sweat glands, the two signals for adjusting better to the heat. This practice keeps the microclimate next to the skin warm and adds to the heat load imposed under externally cool conditions. Dawson et al.[14] used sweat clothing that consisted of a polyester-cotton tracksuit under 100% nylon spray-proof pants and jacket gathered at the wrist and ankles. The jacket was also lined with cotton terry-towelling material which provided extra insulation, and subjects wore a bobble hat of 100% acrylic cloth on their heads. Training in this clothing for 80 minutes each day for one week in temperatures of 10°C induced physiological changes reflecting 'acclimation' and equivalent to those found in another group training for a similar period in hot humid conditions (34°C and 60% relative humidity). Whilst the results showed the effectiveness of sweat clothing for securing acclimation to heat stress, care must be taken if heavy sports clothing is worn on hot days in case the body temperature rises towards hyperthermic levels.

Alternatively, athletes may seek access to an environmental chamber in which heat and humidity can be varied systematically. It is important that periodic bouts of exercise are undertaken in the chamber rather than merely resting in it. Repeated exposures to a sauna or Turkish bath are only partially effective. About 3 hours a week for 2-3 weeks provides a good measure of 'acclimation'. Reilly et al.[15] reported that exercise for 60 minutes at a time, at an intensity corresponding to 70% $\dot{V}O_{2 \text{ max}}$ yielded good results in female hockey players preparing for the Olympic Games. These manoeuvres allow the athlete to experience what the hot conditions to be encountered will feel like.

The warm-weather training camps and the environmental chamber also provide opportunities for inculcating good habits and trying out modifications to normal routines. The athlete in the chamber can become familiarized with drinking during exercise. The coach may learn lessons about how tactics and competitive strategies may need to be altered to cope best with the conditions. The effects of a shortened warm-up, possibly conducted in the shade, can be tested. It may be possible also to identify any individuals intolerant of heat and at risk of heat injury.

HEAT INJURY

Hyperthermia (overheating) and loss of body water (hypohydration) may lead to abnormalities referred to as heat injury. Progressively they can be manifest as muscle cramps, heat exhaustion and heat stroke. They are observed more frequently in individual events such as distance running and cycling than in field games.

Heat cramps are associated with loss of body fluid, particularly when competing in intense heat. Although the body loses electrolytes in sweat, such losses cannot adequately account for cramps occurring. Abnormal spinal reflex activity secondary to local muscle fatigue provides the best explanation of muscle cramps occurring during exercise.[16] Cramps generally coincide with low energy stores and large losses of sodium as well as dehydration. The muscles employed in the exercise are usually affected, especially the leg (upper or lower) and abdominal muscles. Cramps can be stopped by stretching the muscle involved; sometimes massage is effective.

Heat exhaustion is characterized by a core temperature of about 40°C, often seen in unacclimatized individuals. There is a feeling of extreme tiredness, dizziness, breathlessness and tachycardia (increased heart rate). The symptoms may coincide with a reduced sweat loss but usually arise because the skin blood vessels are so dilated that blood flow to vital organs is reduced.

Heat stroke is a true medical emergency. It is characterized by core

---

Box 2.3 Characteristics of heat disorders and injury

Heat cramps:	usually in the unacclimatized
Heat syncope:	general weakness and fatigue; brief loss of consciousness
Heat exhaustion:	dizzy, tired, breathless, reduced sweat loss reduced blood flow to vital organs
	loss of co-ordination
	tachycardia, rise in ventilation
Heat stroke:	confused and irrational state
	skin and core temperature high, skin dry
	pale blue colour
	may hallucinate; may stop sweating
	treat as medical emergency

Box 2.4 Individuals particularly at risk of heat stress

Previous sufferers of heat illness
Unacclimatised individuals
Untrained individuals
Dehydrated individuals
Individuals with high percent body fat
Persons with viral illness
Individuals on medications e.g. diuretics; anti-histamines

---

temperatures of 41°C or higher and dysfunction of the central nervous system. Hypohydration – due to loss of body water in sweat and associated with a high core temperature – can threaten life. Heat stroke is characterized by cessation of sweating, hot and dry flushed skin, total confusion and eventually unconsciousness after collapsing. Treatment is urgently needed to reduce body temperature. There may also be circulatory instability and loss of vasomotor tone as the regulation of blood pressure fails (Box 2.3).

It seems that all racial groups are vulnerable to heat stress: West African athletes, for example, lose their tolerance to heat stress during the rainy season. The rise in body temperature in hot conditions can be the factor that limits performance. Some individuals may be particularly prone to suffering from heat injury (Box 2.4) and caution is advocated in their cases.

AGE AND GENDER

Children differ from adults in a number of important ways with respect to thermoregulatory factors. Children gain (and lose) heat more rapidly than adults do and are more vulnerable than adults in extreme environmental conditions. The exchange of heat with the environment is a function of the ratio between body surface area and body mass. The smaller the individual, the more easily heat is exchanged with the immediate environment. The dimensional exponent for the relationship is 0.67 in adults but differs in children since the surface area to mass ratio of a 10-year-old may be 30% higher than that of an adult. Metabolic heat production is proportional to active muscle mass which is in turn related to body mass. A relatively greater increase in body mass than in body surface area occurs during growth, leading to a decrease in the surface area to body mass ratio.[17]

The physiological mechanisms for exchanging heat with the environment are less well developed in youngsters than in adults. The size of the sweat glands, for example, is directly related to age. There is a correlation between sweat gland size, sweating rate and the cholinergic sensitivity of the glands. Boys show a lower sweating response to a central thermal stimulus than do men. Besides, they display a delayed onset of sweating coupled with a greater rise in skin temperature at a given thermal stress.[15] The favourable surface to mass ratio enables children to rely more on dry heat loss (by radiation, convection and conduction) than by evaporative cooling when exercise is performed in thermoneutral conditions.

Children do not drink enough when they are offered water *ad libitum* in a hot environment. The degree of so-called 'voluntary dehydration' observed in children is similar to that noted in adults. The smaller blood volume in children could accentuate the effects of fluid deficits. The core body temperature of children increases faster than in adults for a given level of hypohydration (defined as percentage loss in body mass) and so prevention of dehydration must be emphasized, even more so than in adult athletes. The availability of beverages palatable to the individual child is therefore important.[18]

Elderly people living at home prefer warmer ambient temperatures than do younger individuals, due to their lower metabolic rate. Yet, they lose some of their capabilities to deal with a high heat load. There is a decrease in blood flow to the skin, reducing the effectiveness of peripheral blood flow as a means of losing heat. There is also a decrease in maximum sweat rate and in insensible perspiration, which is due to a change in the vapour diffusion resistance of the skin with age. The high incidence of fatalities due to hyperthermia among the elderly during the heat wave in Europe in the summer of 2003 reflected the vulnerability of this group to extreme heat. Absence of proper air-conditioning units and existence of cardiovascular morbidities can accentuate the risk. Veteran athletes in good health and with well-trained oxygen transport systems are, in contrast, well equipped for exercise in the heat. Their slower competitive (or training) pace compared to elite athletes means they produce metabolic heat at a comparatively lower rate, thereby attenuating the strain on thermoregulation. The body water content declines with age and there is evidence of a blunted thirst response with ageing.[19] Therefore, attention to fluid replacement should be a priority in veteran sports competitors.

Differences between the sexes in heat exchange are mainly explained by body composition, physique and body surface to volume ratios. These anthropometric factors tend to predominate after differences in fitness and training levels are taken into account. It seems also that the incidence of heat-related injury is roughly similar in men and women, after taking account of ability level and acclimatization.

MONITORING ENVIRONMENTAL TEMPERATURE

The main factors to consider in assessing environmental heat stress are dry bulb temperature, relative humidity, radiant temperature, air velocity and cloud cover. Dry bulb temperature can be measured with a mercury-in-glass thermometer or a hot-wire anemometer whereas relative humidity can be calculated from the data obtained by means of a wet bulb thermometer used in either a sling hygrometer or a Stevenson screen. A hair hygrometer is typically used in laboratory-based studies. The dew point temperature, the point at which the air becomes saturated with water vapour, is a measure of absolute humidity and it can be measured with a whirling hygrometer. Radiant temperature is measured by a globe thermometer inserted into a hollow metal sphere coated with black matt paint. Air velocity can be measured by means of a vane anemometer or an alcohol thermometer coated with polished silver. Cloud cover may provide some intermittent relief to the athlete but will not necessarily protect against ultraviolet solar radiation. More details of the measuring devices and their operations are contained in the classical publication by Bedford.[20]

There have been four main approaches in ergonomics to the evaluation of work under hot conditions:

1. Subjective evaluation of climatic conditions by the subjects
2. Consolidating the physical climatic variables into a single measure
3. Identifying the combinations of climatic variables which produce the same physiological effect, such as the same heart rate and the same core temperature
4. Calculating the energy balance under climatic stress.

A problem for the sports scientist is to find the proper combination of factors to reach an integrated assessment of the environmental heat load. Many equations have been derived for this purpose and three-quarters of a century of research to this end were reviewed by Lee.[21] Most of the formulae incorporate composites of the environmental measures, whereas some, such as the predicted 4-hour sweat rate (P4SR), predict physiological responses from such measures. Probably the most widely used equation in industrial and military establishments has been the WBGT Index, WBGT standing for wet bulb and globe temperature. The US National Institute of Occupational Safety and Health recommended it as the standard heat stress index in 1972. The weightings underline the importance of considering relative humidity:

WBGT = 0.7 WBT + 0.2 GBT + 0.1 DBT
Where: WB represents wet bulb
GB indicates globe
DB represents dry bulb
T indicates temperature.

A comprehensive selection of indices derived in the United Kingdom and the USA was given by Lee.[21] A later development is the Botsball which was validated by Beshir et al.[22] It combines the effects of air temperature, humidity, wind speed and radiation into a single reading. It got its name from its designer, Botsford, and the WBGT can be reliably predicted from the Botsball value if necessary.

Heat stress indices provide a framework for evaluating the risks related to competing in hot conditions and for predicting the casualties. The American College of Sports Medicine[23] set down guidelines for distance races, recommending that events longer than 16 km should not be conducted when the WBGT Index exceeds 28°C. This value is often exceeded in distance races in Europe and in the USA during the summer months, and in many marathon races in Asia and Africa. It is, however, imperative in all cases that the risks be understood and that symptoms of distress are recognized and promptly attended to. The plentiful provision of fluids *en route* and facilities for cooling participants are important precautionary steps. Starting the events in the morning so that competitors finish before the hottest part of the day is another means by which race organizers reduce the incidence of heat-related injuries.

Thermal comfort is achieved as a subjective state of satisfaction within a narrow range of operating thermoequilibrium. The recommended requirements for thermal comfort specified as an international standard (ISO 7730) include that the operative temperature should be 20-24°C, the mean air velocity should not exceed 0.2 m/s and relative humidity should be in the range 30-70%. The percentage of people expressing thermal discomfort if such conditions are met should be less than 10%. It is assumed that the individuals are sedentary but occasionally engaged in light activity.

A comprehensive equation for evaluating the thermal characteristics of the working environment was produced by Fanger.[24] Besides taking the physical features of the environment into consideration, his equation also accounted for activity level, clothing, duration of exposure, and individual differences due to circadian, seasonal, ethnic and gender effects. There are also effects of age but overall these factors balance out. Insensible perspiration in the elderly decreases in proportion to their reduced metabolic rate, so that although less heat is produced there is a corresponding reduction in heat loss compared to young individuals.

OVERVIEW

The core temperature of the body is finely regulated around a narrow physiological range. Humans are homeothermic in that they have the capacity to maintain a relatively constant internal body temperature in the face of high ambient temperatures. The homeostasis is achieved at a cost, in that exercise performance is impaired in conditions of heat stress. The main avenue of losing heat during exercise is by sweating and the resultant dehydration also leads to a fall in performance. Care must be taken to reduce the risk of heat injury. Preparatory measures include acclimation to heat and this adaptation can be achieved relatively quickly in athletes already aerobically trained. Hydration status can be checked daily in groups experiencing warm-weather training. Even in indoor contexts, the appropriate thermal conditions for optimal performance, whether referring to sports performer or worker in a recreation centre, merit consideration. Even at low levels of physical activity, the environmental temperature can have an influence on human comfort and performance.

References

1. Edwards B, Waterhouse J, Reilly T et al. A comparison of the suitabilities of rectal, gut, and insulated axilla temperatures for measurement of the circadian rhythm of core temperature in field studies. Chronobiol Int 2002; 19:579-597
2. Burton AL. Human calorimetry. J Nutr 1935; 9:261-279
3. Ramanathan NL. A new weighting system for mean temperature of the human body. J Appl Physiol 1964; 19:531-533
4. Krustrup P, Mohr M, Bangsbo J. Optimal preparation for the second half: more activities at half-time. The FA Coaches Association Journal 2002; 6(1):60-61
5. Reilly T, Stirling A. Flexibility, warm-up and injuries in mature games players. In: Kinanthropometry IV. Duquet W, Day JAP (eds). London: E and FN Spon, 1993:119-123
6. Astrand PO, Rodahl K. Textbook of work physiology: physiological basis of exercise. 3rd ed. New York: McGraw-Hill, 1986
7. England P, Powers SK, Dodd S et al. The effect of acute thermal dehydration on blood lactate accumulation during incremental exercise. J Sports Sci 1984; 2:105-111
8. Reilly T. Temperature and performance: heat. In: ABC of sports medicine. Harries M, McLatchie G, Williams C, King J (eds). 2nd ed. London: BMJ Books, 2000:68-71
9. Pollock NW, Godfrey RJ, Reilly T. Evaluation of field measures of urine concentration. Med Sci Sports Exerc 1997; 29:S261
10. Hall CJ, Lane AM. Effects of rapid weight loss on mood and performance among amateur boxers. Brit J Sports Med 2001; 35:390-395
11. Hessemer V, Langusch D, Bruck K et al. Effect of slightly lowered body temperature on endurance performance in humans. J Appl Physiol 1984; 57:1731-1737
12. Olschewski H, Bruck K. Thermoregulatory, cardiovascular and muscular factors related to exercise after precooling. J Appl Physiol 1988; 64:803-811
13. Drust B, Cable NT, Reilly T. Investigation of the effects of pre-cooling on the physiological responses to soccer-specific intermittent exercise. Europ J Appl Physiol 2000; 81:11-17
14. Dawson B, Pyke FS, Morton AR. Improvements in heat tolerance induced by interval running training in the heat and in sweat clothing in cool conditions. J Sports Sci 1989; 7:189-203

5. Reilly T, Maughan RJ, Budgett R et al. The acclimatisation of international athletes. In: Contemporary ergonomics. Robertson SA (ed) London: Taylor and Francis, 1997:136-141

16. Schwellnus MP, Derman EW, Noakes TD. Aetiology of skeletal muscle 'changes' during exercise. A novel hypothesis. J Sports Sci 1997; 15:277-285

17. Falk B. Temperature regulation. In: Paediatric exercise science and medicine. Armstrong N, von Mechelen W (eds). Oxford: Oxford University Press, 2000:223-239

18. Bar-Or O. The young athlete: some physiological considerations. J Sports Sci 1995; 13:531-533

19. Ainslie PN, Campbell IT, Frayn KN et al. Energy balance, metabolism, hydration and performance during strenuous hill walking: the effect of age. J Appl Physiol 2002; 93:714-723

20. Bedford T. Environmental warmth and its measurement. Medical Research Council War Memorandum no 17. HMSO: London, 1946

21. Lee DHK. Seventy five years of searching for a heat index. Environ Res 1980; 22:331-356

22. Beshir MY, Ramsey JD, Burford CL. Threshold values for the Botsball: a field study of occupational heat. Ergonomics 1982; 25:247-254

23. American College of Sports Medicine. Position stand: The prevention of thermal injuries during distance running. Med Sci Sports Exerc 1987; 19:529-533

24. Fanger PO. Thermal comfort. New York: McGraw-Hill, 1970

Chapter 3

Exercise in the cold

CHAPTER CONTENTS

Introduction 33
Thermoregulation and the cold 35
Coping with cold conditions 38
Water immersion 40
Cold pathologies 43
Adaptation to cold 44

Monitoring environmental cold stress 45
Preparing for cold conditions 47
Overview 47

INTRODUCTION

Besides the so-called winter sports, many games are played in conditions which are often near-freezing. Furthermore, recreational activities such as hill walking may entail exposure to low environmental temperatures and there is a risk of immersion in very cold water when boating accidents occur. Core and muscle temperatures may fall and, when exercise is performed in the cold, the quality of performance can be increasingly affected; consciousness is impaired as core temperature drops to its lower safe limit of about 35°C. Hypothermia is life-threatening and the body's heat gain mechanisms are designed to arrest the decline in body temperature.

With the fall in limb temperature arising from cutaneous vasoconstriction, motor performance deteriorates. Muscle power output is reduced by about 3% for every 1°C fall in muscle temperature below normal. Along with the drop in muscular strength and power output as the temperature in the muscle falls, conduction velocity of nerve impulses to the muscles is slowed. Sensitivity of muscle spindles also declines and manual dexterity is impaired. Despite very low ambient air temperatures, limb temperatures can be preserved by wearing appropriate gloves.

The normal skin temperature is about 33°C, averaged throughout the whole body. Extreme thermal discomfort is felt when this mean value falls below 25°C. Lower values can be tolerated in the extremities but when the skin temperature drops below 23°C, limb movements become clumsy; finger

Table 3.1 Critical temperatures for different biological tissues[2]

Tissue	Temperature (°C)
Nerves	20
Receptors	10
Joints	24
Muscles	
Dynamic force	38
Dynamic endurance	28
Static force	28–38
Static endurance	28
Skin	
Local	15
Mean	?
Core	?

dexterity is severely affected at skin temperatures around 15°C and performance of fine manipulative tasks is impaired. The tactile sensitivity of the fingers deteriorates to the extent that an impact on the skin at 20°C has to be six times greater than normal for usual sensations to be registered.[1] The synovial fluid in the joints becomes more viscous as its temperature falls, thereby increasing joint stiffness. These changes render the individual more vulnerable to accidents if exposure to the cold is continued.

It seems that mean skin temperature and core body temperature play a minor role in affecting manual dexterity in comparison with the local temperature in the hands and fingers. Loss of dexterity is not inevitable as long as joint temperature exceeds 24°C, nerve temperature is above 20°C and local skin temperature is greater than 15°C.[2] A nerve block occurs at skin temperatures around 6°C and nerve temperatures of 10°C when there is no further conduction of nerve signals to the fingers (see Table 3.1).

According to the study of Galloway and Maughan,[3] an ambient temperature of about 11°C is optimal for endurance on a cycle ergometer, close to the value of 14°C for distance runners. Exercise to exhaustion at 70% $\dot{V}O_{2\ max}$ was reduced from 93.5 min to 81.4 and 81.2 min when the environmental temperature was changed to 4°C and 20°C respectively. A further decline in performance was observed when the temperature was raised to 30°C.

There is a wide range of sports in which participants are exposed to cold. The skier on the chair-lift may be cooled while ascending the mountain for the next bout of activity. The recreational hill walker can experience vastly different weather conditions even within a single day. The experienced adventurer is programmed to anticipate the worst climatic conditions.

Leaders of expeditions, whether on land or sea, must plan their itineraries carefully to avoid disaster. Sailors acknowledge their vulnerability to cold, wet and windy conditions and survival may depend on forecasting impending adversities. Some of these difficulties are considered in this chapter, along with the human's capabilities to cope with them.

THERMOREGULATION AND THE COLD

The thermoregulatory responses to cold are initiated by the 'heat gain centre' in the posterior hypothalamus. Cutaneous inputs are relayed to the 'centre' from cold receptors, which sense the environmental temperature to which the skin is exposed. A generalized peripheral vasoconstriction of the cutaneous circulation, mediated by the sympathetic nervous system, displaces blood from the shell to the core in response to cold. The decrease in peripheral blood flow reduces heat loss to the environment but the changes in blood flow are not uniform throughout the body. Flow to the fingers may decline by a factor of 40 compared with normal whereas, with no vasoconstrictor fibres to the scalp, blood flow to the head remains unaltered. Consequently heat loss through the head contributes towards hypothermia in cold conditions; covering the head offers protection.

The shift of blood centrally from the cutaneous circulation increases the temperature gradient between the core and the shell. The reduction in skin temperature in turn decreases the gradient between the skin and the environment and protects against large losses of heat to the environment (see Figure 3.1). Superficial veins are cooled further in that blood returning from the limbs is diverted from the superficial blood vessels to the venae comitantes that lie adjacent to the main arteries. This diversion reduces heat loss since the arterial blood is thereby cooled by the venous return almost immediately it enters the limb by means of counter-current heat exchange.

If the environment is extremely cold, there may be a delayed vasodilation of the blood vessels in the skin, which alternates with intense vasoconstriction in cycles of 15-30 minutes and leads to excessive heat loss (see Figure 3.2). This oscillation has been described as a hunting reaction in the quest for an appropriate skin temperature to achieve the best combination of gradients between the core, shell and environment. The vasodilation may be the result of accumulated vasoactive metabolites arising from increased anaerobic metabolism in local tissues that is associated with the reduced blood flow. It seems that the smooth muscle located in the walls of peripheral blood vessels is paralyzed at temperatures of 10°C; as the muscles cannot then respond to noradrenaline released by vasoconstrictor nerves, the muscles relax to cause a return of blood flow through the vessels, thus completing the cycle.[3] The mechanism may be a way of reducing the processes of frostbite, although the vasodilation itself increases the loss of heat from the digits. This alternation of high and low blood flow to local tissue produced by ice-pack application is exploited in the treatment of sports injuries by physiotherapists. The phenomenon is also well recognized by

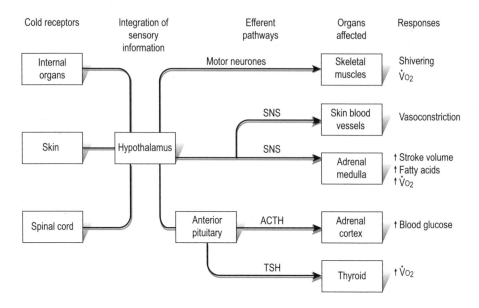

Figure 3.1 Regulation of thermal responses protecting against hypothermia

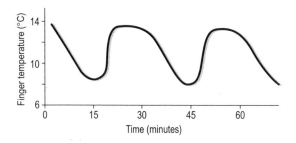

Figure 3.2 The phenomenon of cold vasodilation (modified from Keatinge, 1969)

runners and cyclists if they train in cold conditions without wearing gloves; initially the fingers are white as a result of vasoconstriction but they become a ruddy colour as blood enters the digits in increased volumes.

Blood flow to the skin may also be influenced by alcohol, which has a vasodilator effect. Though alcohol can make a person feel more comfortable when exposed to cold, it will increase heat loss and so may endanger the individual. Consequently, drinking alcohol is not recommended when staying outdoors overnight in inclement weather conditions and the customary hip-flask of whisky (or lunch-time glasses of wine) serves no useful protective function for recreational skiers or mountaineers. It may further compound the body water losses occurring as a result of cold diuresis.

This physiological response is secondary to the vasoconstriction induced by the cold and the resulting redistribution of body fluids to the central circulation from the periphery. Exercise minimizes cold-induced vasoconstriction whilst the decrease in blood flow through the kidneys blunts the diuresis induced by the cold. The overall result is that the effect is self-limiting.

Shivering is a response of the body's autonomic nervous system to falling core temperature. It constitutes involuntary activity of skeletal muscles to generate metabolic heat. Shivering tends to be intermittent and even persists during exercise if the intensity is insufficient to maintain core temperature. It may be evident during stoppages in activity, such as in hill walkers resting whilst taking a snack in open unsheltered conditions. Shivering represents an early warning of the body's struggle to maintain heat balance. The energy for shivering emanates from adenosine triphosphate, being the source of fuel for muscle contractions. As no mechanical work is done in shivering, practically all of the energy released contributes to the generation of heat. Generalized shivering incorporates the major muscle groups of the body and can increase metabolic rate by a factor of five times the resting value.

Basal heat production may be elevated by means of the neuroendocrine system in conditions of long-term cold exposure. The hypothalamus stimulates the pituitary gland to release hormones that affect other target organs, notably the thyroid and adrenal glands. The resultant elevation in metabolism will persist throughout a sojourn, the metabolic rate at rest being greater in cold than in temperate climates and elevated over that of tropical residents. Adrenaline and adrenocortical hormones may also cause a slight increase in metabolism, though the combined hormonal effects are still relatively modest. Brown fat, so-called because of its iron-containing cytochromes active in oxidative processes, is a potential source of thermogenesis. This form of fat is located primarily in and around the kidneys and adjacent to the great vessels, beneath the shoulder blades and along the spine. It is evident in abundance in infants, in whom shivering mechanisms are poorly developed but its stores decline during growth and development. Its high metabolic rate has been presented as an explanation for why some individuals fail to increase body weight despite appearing to overeat, though this point is highly contentious.

There is some evidence that cold may increase carbohydrate utilisation, possibly mediated by reduced blood flow to skeletal muscles.[5] Whereas increased noradrenaline would be expected to promote lipolysis, there seems to be an uncoupling of the availability and the utilisation of fats when the environmental temperature goes below 5°C.[6,7] Maintaining normal levels of liver and muscle glycogen may be important in protecting individuals against the cold: hypoglycaemia inhibits shivering, thereby reducing involuntary metabolic heat production.[8]

The reduction of blood flow to the skin and subcutaneous adipose tissue converts the body's 'shell' into an insulated buffer zone which protects the core and its vital organs against the cold. The skeletal muscles can also provide significant insulation when they are relatively underperfused with blood at rest. However, they lose this insulating property during exercise as blood enters the active muscles.

COPING WITH COLD CONDITIONS

Cold is less problematic than heat, since the body may be protected against exposure to the ambient environment. The microclimate surrounding the skin is critical; it may be maintained by appropriate choice of clothing. Behaviourally, individuals might respond to cold by maintaining a high work-rate. Alternatively, games players may be spared exposure to cold by training in available indoor facilities.

The insulating capacity of clothing refers to its ability to retain body heat and is expressed in clothing (CLO) units. The amount of insulation provided by ordinary business dress is equal to 1 CLO unit, whereby the individual is comfortable at 21°C with low air velocity and relative humidity. At the environmental extremes of the north and south-polar regions, the clothing for Eskimos provides about 10-12 CLO units. The insulating properties of clothing are reduced when the clothing gets wet, because water is a far worse insulator than air.

Clothing of natural fibre (cotton or wool) is preferable to synthetic material in cold and in cold-wet conditions. The clothing should be windproof as well as waterproof. Adequate insulation is best achieved by using a number of layers underneath the outer garment. The clothing should allow sweat produced during exercise in these conditions, as well as any build up of condensation, to flow through the garment. The best material is permeable to moisture vapour and will allow sweat to flow out through the cells of the garment whilst preventing water droplets from penetrating the clothing from the outside. If the fabric becomes saturated with water or sweat, it loses its insulation qualities and in cold-wet conditions the body loses extra heat and then core temperature may quickly drop. The clothing found on the fatalities reported by Pugh[9] for the Four Inns walking disaster had lost 90% of its insulatory properties. In extreme cold conditions, climbers use two fleece layers of trousers and tops or jacket, and a further 'down suit' over them. The ensemble of garments must be flexible for taking off or putting on and permit unhindered movement. A thin neoprene face mask may be used for facial protection and a thick balaclava to prevent heat loss through the head. The scalp has no vasoconstrictive fibres to its blood vessels and so is slow to respond to any direct effect of cooling.[1] As 25% of the heat produced may be lost through the head, the importance of protecting it against the cold is obvious.

Hypothermia has long been recognised as a serious risk in hill walking and fell running, often leading to fatal consequences. Hill walkers may operate at 30 to 55% of maximal oxygen uptake, depending on the terrain. When exercising at this intensity, metabolic heat production is usually sufficient to offset heat loss. Even if weather conditions are adverse, rectal temperatures of

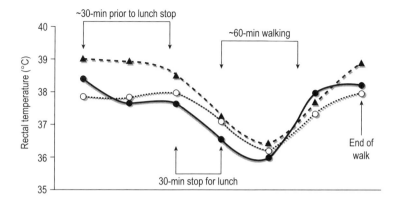

Figure 3.3 The apparent fall in temperature in hill-walkers after stopping for 30 min to eat lunch (from Ainslie et al., 2001)

39°C have been reported, the well insulated clothing preventing heat loss. Once the walker fatigues and starts to slow or stop completely, the rate of heat production falls dramatically. This change in activity alone predisposes to heat loss[8] and upsets the balance between heat production and its dissipation. The critical point in adverse weather is when participants stop to rest or for food and drink in the open (see Figure 3.3).

Athletes training in the cold should keep the trunk area of the body well insulated. Warm undergarments may be worn beneath a full tracksuit. Dressing in layers is advised: outer layers can be discarded as body temperature rises and if ambient temperature gets warmer. Wearing a suitable cap offers protection against the large heat losses that would otherwise occur through the head. When layers of clothing are worn, the outer layer should be capable of resisting both wind and rain. The inner layer should provide insulation and also wick moisture from the skin to promote heat loss by evaporation. Polypropylene and cotton fishnet thermal underwear, having good insulation and wicking properties, is suitable to wear next to the skin.

The best way of protecting the hands and feet is to maintain core body temperature so that there is continued peripheral blood flow to keep the limbs warm. The hands and feet cool quickly following vasoconstriction because of their relatively high surface area. Gloves and footwear help to insulate the limbs but will not keep them warm if body temperature has fallen. Fingerless mittens are superior to gloves in providing insulation because of the decrease in area of the surface that is exposed.

Strategies for coping with cold conditions must integrate a behavioural approach with appropriate use of cold-protective clothing. Immediately prior to competing in the cold, games players should stay warm. A thorough warm-up (performed indoors if possible) is recommended. Cold increases the risk of muscle injury in sports involving anaerobic efforts; warm-up exercises afford some protection against injury, particularly muscle tears. Competitors may need to wear more clothing than they normally do during matches or when competing in individual sports.

Whilst a majority of the world's population may reside in warm or temperate climates, many people manage to live their lives in extreme cold. (The lowest temperature recorded in recent years in an area of human habitation was -71.2°C in Oymyakon, Siberia whilst a temperature of -89°C was recorded in mid-East Antarctica in July 1983.) They do so by a combination of lifestyle factors, complemented by physiological adaptations. Suitably protected, they can tolerate ambient temperatures of -50°C and colder. In effect, they are not actually exposed to extremes of temperature since the microclimate next to the skin's surface is kept warm by air trapped within and underneath their clothing. It is also essential that the domestic accommodation affords protection against hostile weather conditions. Such protection is exemplified in the igloos of the Eskimos, the air trapped in their walls providing perfect insulation for the dwellers.

Cold injuries suffered by residents of the British Antarctic over the 10-year period 1986-1995 included 58 cases of frostbite, two cases of hypothermia and one case of so-called trench-foot. The annual incidence of cold injury was only 66 per 1000 people.[12] The face and ears were the most common locations of superficial frostbite, occurring in roughly half of the cases in mean ambient temperatures of -21°C (range – 0.3°C to -42.5°C). In the five years 1991-1995 in Alaska, there were 327 people hospitalized for cold-related injuries. Of these, hypothermia accounted for 46% of the total admissions, whilst frostbite in the feet amounted to 42% of cases.[13]

Cold weather conditions are also implicated in injuries to hill walkers.[14] Accidental hypothermia can occur due to inadequacy of clothing or footwear, the rapid drop in core temperature if activity is halted or getting lost as bad weather closes in. Typically walkers become dehydrated and incur a negative energy balance of some 7 MJ as a consequence of a day's activity on the hills. It is therefore not surprising that almost two-thirds of injuries have been reported to occur towards the end of walks sustained for 6-8 hours.[14]

WATER IMMERSION

Water has a 25-fold greater thermal conductivity than air and a volume-specific heat capacity 3500 times greater,[11] and therefore heat is readily exchanged with the environment when the human body is immersed. The preferred water temperature for inactive individuals is 32-33°C, for those learning to swim it is about 30°C, for active swimmers 27°C and for competitive swimmers 25°C. The reason for these differential values is the metabolic heat produced during swimming, which is a function of the exercise intensity. High humidity in swimming pools protects the swimmers against heat loss when out of the water but is not optimal for the comfort of spectators. Air temperature in the region 28-30°C accentuates this discomfort.

The greater the swimming intensity the lower is the water temperature for greatest efficiency. This relationship is influenced by the physique and body composition of the swimmer. Lean swimmers are unable to maintain $\dot{V}O_{2\,max}$ at a water temperature of 26°C whereas fatter subjects show a similar failure at 18°C. The muscle mass complements the subcutaneous adipose tissue layers in insulating the body and prolongs exposure time in accidental immersion. The adipose tissue is relatively underperfused; fat has a thermal conductivity half that of skeletal muscle and one-third that of blood, so the thickness of the subcutaneous layer determines the heat flow from the body to the water.

Muscle function is adversely influenced by cold water immersion, grip strength in water as low as 2°C falling quickly to half the normal value. The decline in muscle strength that occurs with time on exposure to water at low temperature is referred to as the 'muscle fatigue curve'. Muscle fatigue curves are detrimentally affected by immersion for 8 minutes at 10°C but complete recovery occurs within 40 minutes of exposure. As muscle temperature falls below 27°C, muscle spindles respond at only 50% of normal to a standard stimulus, thereby affecting motor co-ordination. The fall in finger temperature will be even more pronounced, severely impairing manual dexterity.

Few people accidentally immersed in ice-cold water will live for more than a few minutes. The limited survival time in these low temperatures is due to the cold-shock response. Ice-cold water induces a peripheral vasoconstriction, elevation in heart rate and increased cardiac output. Systolic pressure is raised as a result, as high as 180 mmHg. There is an immediate hyperventilation, which disturbs the normal coupling of respiration and muscular activity and the results are inhalation of water and failure to swim. Further, the duration of the normal breath-hold is reduced. The hyperventilation causes a marked respiratory alkalosis leading to a reduction in cerebral blood flow and resultant disorientation. Finally the hyperventilation induces a strong feeling of dyspnoea and may indicate panic. All these factors increase the risk of drowning in water at a low temperature.

Golden and Tipton[6] considered that body cooling and onset of hypothermia increase the likelihood of water aspiration and drowning before death from hypothermia. They outlined the sequence of events that threaten survival of people accidentally immersed in open water. First, the cold-shock response could cause cardiovascular problems or even drowning. Second, cooling of muscle and peripheral nerves could cause incapacitation and result in drowning. Third, incapacitation and drowning will be a direct result of hypothermia. Death might also result from cardiac arrest due to hypothermia.

In ocean temperatures not quite ice-cold, survival times in water are greatly extended in individuals with high levels of adiposity. The subcutaneous layers of adipose tissue provide insulation for the organs within the body's core and attenuate heat loss to the environment. It seems

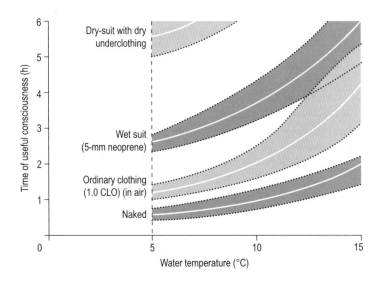

Figure 3.4 Survival times in water of different temperatures when wearing clothing differing in insulation properties. The influence of clothing on survival times increases at temperatures >10°C[11]

that ultra-endurance swimmers, such as those successfully crossing the English Channel, are self-selected and rarely include lean individuals. Survival times in cold water are increased by wearing dry suits or wet suits. The former are designed to keep the body dry whereas the latter allow through a minimal amount of water, which is then heated by the body and, after equalizing with skin temperature and becoming part of the boundary layer next to the skin, prevents further heat loss from it. Wet suits are usually made of closed-cell neoprene 3-6 mm in thickness and need to fit closely for effectiveness. The protective value of different clothing at temperatures from 5 to 15°C as expressed in time of useful consciousness is shown in Figure 3.4. The wearing of a wet suit increases survival time at 5°C by a factor of six whilst the time is extended ten-fold by the use of a dry suit. For greatest effectiveness, these suits should cover the arms, in view of the fact that more heat is lost from the arms compared to the legs when each limb is exercised at the same absolute oxygen uptake.[17]

The cold-shock response is likely to cause death within 5-10 minutes on accidental exposure to ice-cold water. Good health and physical fitness are helpful in surviving these initial crises. Swimming to safety will only be possible if the shore is close by and few will be able to cover 100 m. Survival times are extended considerably in warmer water between 10 and 15°C. The risk of dying in the water is associated with both cooling of the limb muscles, resulting in physical incapacitation and drowning as a consequence, and loss of consciousness due to the fall in whole-body temperature. Physical

Box 3.1 Selected effects of cold on human performance

Peripheral vasoconstriction increases

Metabolism rises

Shivering (periodic)

Muscle spindle sensitivity falls

Nerve conduction velocity - delayed

Manual dexterity falls

Muscle strength/power falls

Accidents rise

incapacitation would occur in an individual attempting to cling to wreckage, for example. The fall in core temperature would occur ultimately in those who chose to swim in the cold water, although fatter individuals would last longer than would lean ones.[18]

COLD PATHOLOGIES

Hypothermia refers to a fall in core temperature to a level where life is threatened. Early symptoms of hypothermia include shivering, fatigue, losses of strength, motor co-ordination and the ability to sustain work-rate (see Box 3.1). Diuresis accompanies a prolonged exposure to cold. Once fatigue develops, shivering may decrease and the condition worsens. Later symptoms include collapse, stupor and loss of consciousness. Individuals who are unable to sustain a work-rate of sufficient intensity to keep themselves in thermal equilibrium in extreme cold are particularly vulnerable.

The cold stress leading to hypothermia is progressively manifested by an enlargement of the area of the body shell, whereas the area of the core becomes smaller and smaller. The result is that the core temperature ultimately reaches a dangerously low level. A core temperature of 34.5°C is usually taken as indicative of grave hypothermic risk, although there is no absolute consensus of a critical end-point. Keatinge et al.[19] considered that a core temperature of 34.3°C, recorded in a Russian participant swimming in water below 11°C, was not a threat to life when facilities to re-warm in a sauna were immediately available. Body temperatures below 32°C cause a progressive risk of spontaneous ventricular fibrillation and death. The exact value of hypothalamic temperature that would be fatal is also subject to controversy. In cases of severe hypothermia, there is a risk of subsequent circulatory, respiratory and renal failure. An immediate aim must be to get

Table 3.2 Cold pathologies

Cold exhaustion:	lowered body temperature
	hypoglycaemia
	cerebral function falls
	motor co-ordination falls
	confusion increases
	accidents rise
Frostbite:	skin temperature–freezing point
	intense local vasoconstriction
	contact with cold material

the victim to shelter, provide hot fluid and extra clothing and consider means of evacuation to hospital.

Frostbite refers to a destruction of superficial tissues that can occur when the temperature in the nose, fingers or toes falls below freezing. At -1°C ice crystals are formed in those tissues. The first sign of frostbite is a cloudy white appearance of the skin, indicating that the skin is frozen. Warming the affected tissue provides adequate treatment at this stage. The colour of the surface flesh appears black when advanced frostbite sets in. As blood flow can no longer be restored, the result can be manifest as a gangrenous extremity such as experienced by mountaineers in icy conditions when their gloves or boots fail to provide adequate thermal insulation (see Table 3.2). Recent clinical experience is that amputation of damaged tissue is not a necessary consequence of frostbite and prognosis tends to be more optimistic than thought in previous decades. Tissue from intact areas may be used for reconstruction, for example when the nose is lost due to frostbite. Nevertheless, even mild forms of frostbite can be extremely painful for weeks after recovery due to formation of blisters and damage to skin layers.

ADAPTATION TO COLD

Acclimatization to cold is less pronounced than to heat; behavioural and proper clothing strategies can safeguard individuals in cold environments. Some physiological adaptations do occur, starting with the first experience of cold conditions.

Thyroxine increases metabolic rate within 5-6 hours of cold exposure. The elevated thyroxine output persists throughout the sojourn. Adrenaline and adrenocorticoid hormones contribute to the increase in metabolic rate. A thermogenic reaction to the secretion of noradrenaline develops from prolonged exposure but the main response of habituated individuals is peripheral vasoconstriction in the cold.

Physiological adaptations in fishermen occupationally exposed to cold water include changes in the typical acute responses of the circulation to cold exposure. Vasoconstriction in cooled blood vessels of the hands and feet is intermittently reversed to a pattern of cold-induced vasodilation. The vasodilation occurs more frequently and lasts longer with acclimatization to cold, and there is a decrease in the initial vasoconstrictor response.[20] These peripheral vascular changes are accompanied by a reduction in the central blood pressure response to cold exposure; this mechanism allows the so-called 'sport hardeners' dwelling near the Arctic Circle to swim in icy waters for short-term recreational purposes. The peripheral vascular mechanisms for facilitating tolerance of cold may also have a habituation element, allowing the Bushmen of the Kalahari desert and the Aboriginals of the Australian outback to sleep outdoors at night in very low ambient temperatures. By restricting peripheral circulation, they are able to endure cold conditions that would seriously endanger visiting tourists if similarly exposed.

A habituation effect also seems to reduce the cold-shock response in water. Upon repeated immersions the decrease in minute ventilation ($\dot{V}E$) is reduced to below one-third of its initial response and subjects display little distress on immersion. Even five 2-minute immersions in cold water can decrease the cold-shock response by half, the habituation effect persisting for up to 12 months. Short exposures to a cold shower have a similar but less marked effect.[11]

The added protection against the cold offered by physiological adaptations is likely to be inadequate for the visitor unless behavioural adjustments are also made. In this respect preparation and planning for exposure to the cold are essentials. It is important also to learn from the experience of others as this information may be the difference between survival and death. Indeed, Keatinge et al.[19] found that experienced swimmers during a marathon relay in water at 9-11°C were able to assess subjectively when to leave the water as the body temperature approached hazardous levels.

MONITORING ENVIRONMENTAL COLD STRESS

Existence of good rescue facilities is no excuse for climbing parties to take risks in inclement weather. Early warning systems used by rangers on mountainsides must be heeded if they are to be effective and this inevitably means consumer education. Otherwise, the safety of the rescue team in addition to that of the climbing party may be jeopardized if weather conditions further deteriorate. Assessment of the risk involves some calculations of the magnitude of cold stress.

On the mountainside the wind velocity may be the most influential factor in cooling the body so that the ambient temperature alone would grossly underestimate the prevailing risk. The wind-chill index designed by Siple and Passel,[21] and widely used by mountaineers and skiers, provides a method of comparing different combinations of temperature and wind speed (Box 3.2). The values calculated correspond to a caloric scale for rate of heat loss per unit body surface area; they are then converted into a sensation scale ranging from hot (about 80) through cool (400) to bitterly cold (1200) and on to a value at which exposed flesh freezes within 60 seconds. The cooling

Box 3.2 Wind chill formula for calculating heat loss

$Ko = (100V + 10.5 - V)^{0.5} * (33 - T)$

Ko = heat loss in kcal/h
V = wind velocity in m/s
T = environmental temperature in °C
10.5 = a constant
33 = assumed normal skin temperature in °C

Box 3.3 Rating scale for subjective sensation of cold

2	Comfortably warm
1	
0	Neutral
-1	
-2	Comfortably cold
-3	
-4	Uncomfortably cold
-5	
-6	Cold
-7	
-8	Very cold
-9	
-10	Very very cold

effects of combinations of certain temperatures and wind speeds are expressed as 'temperature equivalents' and are estimated by means of a nomogram. Use of the wind-chill index enables sojourners to evaluate the magnitude of cold stress and take appropriate precautions. Wet conditions can exacerbate cold stress, especially if the clothing worn is not waterproof or begins to lose its insulation. Attention to safety may be even more important in water sports since, apart from the risk of drowning, body heat is lost much more rapidly in water than in air.

For indoor environments, an alternative approach is needed. Holmer[22] developed a heat exchange model for the assessment of thermal stress in cold environments. The model integrates the effects of air temperature, mean radiant temperature, humidity, air velocity and metabolic rate. He specified the required clothing insulation (Ireq, i.e. insulation required) against excessive dry heat loss for defined levels of physiological strain and calculated time limits for exposure at given levels of clothing insulation. As thermal equilibrium can be achieved at different levels of thermoregulatory strain and is defined by mean skin temperature, skin wettedness (due to sweating) and change in body heat content, two levels of required insulation were suggested:

- Ireq min – represents the minimal insulation needed to maintain thermal equilibrium at a subnormal level; in other words, the highest admissible body cooling during physical activity
- Ireq neutral – defines the insulation required to maintain thermal equilibrium at a normal level.

These standards were designed for occupational purposes. Nevertheless the approach may be useful in testing sports clothing for outdoor conditions, especially where extreme cold may be encountered.

Subjective sensations can be of value in monitoring responses to cold. An example of a rating scale for assessment of general cold sensation is shown in Box 3.3. A limitation is that it fails to take into account local or unilateral cooling, as might occur indoors when exposed to a draught.

PREPARING FOR COLD CONDITIONS

It is important to plan in detail for expeditions in cold conditions. For short-term exposures weather forecasts are helpful. As the weather conditions can change quite quickly, on the seas or the mountainside for example, the worst of the possible conditions should be catered for. Expedition leaders have particular responsibilities for calculating necessary provisions, clothing and loads to be transported or carried. In inclement weather when conditions deteriorate, original plans need to be modified to reduce risks of cold exposure and hypothermia.

For many outdoor recreation participants, portable housing can ensure against hypothermia, especially in case of overnight stays on the mountainside. Besides the major advances in design of boots and clothing for the cold, the reliability and durability of tents have much improved. A similar systematic improvement is noted in the provision of first aid and rescue services for outdoor pursuits. The availability of good rescue facilities should never be an excuse for expeditions to take risks in inclement weather.

OVERVIEW

Cold constitutes a potential threat to life, especially when the weather changes rapidly and the individual is inadequately prepared for it. Cold conditions are to be anticipated in all outdoor winter sports, in recreational excursions to wilderness areas and at altitude. Preparation entails a choice of appropriate clothing and footwear, adequate provisions and training to construct shelter if accidentally isolated. Whilst there is some evidence of an acclimatization to cold, the most effective means of protection against hypothermia is behavioural in nature.

As heat is exchanged much more easily in water than in air, there are many water-sports activities in which accidental immersion places the participant at risk. Wearing a life-jacket and full clothing provides some amount of protection but survival in cold water is also dependent on individual factors. Elderly individuals are less likely to survive accidents at sea than are their younger counterparts and lean individuals lose heat rapidly in such circumstances. Channel swimmers tend to be muscular and to possess large subcutaneous adipose tissue deposits which help insulate them against the cold during their long-distance attempts.

Rescue crews, whether operating on the mountains or on the seas, may have to expose themselves to risk when called upon in emergencies. They require specialist skills in diagnosing symptoms of hypothermia and related problems. They also need to have a sound knowledge of appropriate treatment and must often make life-saving decisions upon locating their victim. For the latter, the experience of rescue can itself be traumatic, especially if serious injury has occurred to themselves or their colleagues.

References

1. Reilly T, Cable NT. Thermoregulation. In: Kinanthropometry and exercise physiology laboratory manual. Vol 2. Eston RG, Reilly T (eds). London: Routledge, 2001:193-210
2. Heus R, Daanen HAM, Havenith G. Physiological criteria for functioning of hands in the cold. Appl Ergon 1995; 26:5-13
3. Galloway SDR, Maughan RJ. Effects of ambient temperature on the capacity to perform prolonged cycle exercise in man. Med Sci Sports Exerc 1997; 29:1240-1249
4. Keatinge WR. Survival in cold water. Oxford: Blackwell, 1969
5. Samra JS, Simpson EJ, Clark ML et al. Effects of epinephrine infusion on adipose tissue: interaction between blood flow and metabolism. Amer J Physiol 1996; 271: E834-E839
6. Vallerand AL, Zamecrik J, Jones PJH et al. Cold stress increases lipolysis, FFA, Ra and TG/FFA cycling in humans. Aviat Space Environ Med 1999; 70:42-50
7. Layden JD, Patterson MJ, Nimmo MA. Effect of reduced ambient temperature on fat utilization during submaximal exercise. Med Sci Sports Exerc 2002; 34:774-799
8. Tipton MJ, Golden F st C. Immersion in cold water: effects on performance and safety. In: Oxford textbook of sports medicine, 2nd edn. Harries M, Williams C, Stanish WD et al (eds). Oxford: Oxford Medical Publishers, 1998: 241-254
9. Pugh LGCE. Cold stress and muscular exercise, with special reference to accidental hypothermia. BMJ 1967; 2:333-337
10. Ainslie PN, Campbell IT, Frayn KN et al. Physiological aspects of hill-walking. In: Contemporary Ergonomics. Hanson MA (ed). London: Taylor and Francis, 2001:8-14
11. Golden F, Tipton M. Essentials of sea survival. Champaign, Il Human Kinetics 2002
12. Cattermole TJ. The epidemiology of cold injury in Antarctica. Aviat Space Environ Med 1999; 70:135-140
13. Conway GA, Husberg BJ. Cold-related non-fatal injuries in Alaska. Am J Ind Med (Suppl) 1999; 1:39-41

14. Ainslie P, Reilly T. Physiology of accidental hypothermia in the mountains : a forgotten story. Brit J Sports Med 2003; 37: 548-550.
15. Ainslie PN, Campbell IT, MacLaren DPM et al. Characteristic activities and injuries of hill-walkers. In: Contemporary ergonomics. McCabe PT (ed). London: Taylor and Francis, 2002:167-171
16. Noakes TD. Exercise and the cold. Advances in sport, leisure and ergonomics. Reilly T, Greeves J (eds). London: Routledge, 2002:13-31
17. Toner MM, Sawka MN, Pandolf KB. Thermal responses during arm and leg and combined arm-leg exercise in water. J Appl Physiol 1984; 52:1557-1564
18. Tipton M, Eglin C, Genner M et al. Immersion deaths and deterioration in swimming performance in cold water: a volunteer trial. Lancet 1999; 354:626-629
19. Keatinge WR, Khartchenko M, Lando N et al. Hypothermia during sports swimming in water below 11°C. Brit J Sports Med 2001; 35:352-353
20. Stroud MA. Exercise in the cold. Sports Exerc Inj 1997; 3:25-30
21. Siple PA, Passel CF. Measurement of dry atmosphere cooling in sub-freezing temperatures. Proc Am Phil Soc 1945; 89:177-199
22. Holmer I. Assessment of cold stress in terms of required clothing insulation – Ireq. Int J Ind Erg 1988; 3:159-166

Chapter 4

Altitude stress and hypoxia

CHAPTER CONTENTS

Introduction 51
Physiological background 52
Extreme altitude 55
High altitudes 58
Moderate altitudes 60
Effects of moderate altitude on
   exercise performance 61

Acute adaptations 63
Metabolic adaptations 65
Altitude training camps 66
Simulated altitude 68
Non-responders to altitude training 69
Overview 70

INTRODUCTION

The dream to ascend higher than ever before has been a historical human aspiration that is exemplified in the fable of Icarus whose wings of wax melted as he flew too near the sun. The quest is reflected in sports such as ballooning, parachuting, flying and the pinnacle of mountaineering achievement, the conquest of Mount Everest. Research in aviation medicine has contributed to the understanding of how the human reacts in the event of abrupt decreases in ambient pressure and the adaptations that occur so that humans can tolerate these inhospitable conditions.

The recreational climber or skier makes sojourns to moderate altitude where the environmental stress is not so extreme. Similarly, many sports participants now engage in exercise at altitude; these range from mountaineers and rock climbers to recreational skiers and trekkers on activity holidays. Additionally, sport competitions are occasionally held at altitude; these have included the 1968 Olympic Games in Mexico City and subsequently the World Cup soccer tournaments there in 1970 and 1986. Rugby Union teams preparing for the World Cup in South Africa in 1995 had to consider the prospects of playing some matches at altitude and cyclists attempting to qualify for the 1996 Olympic Games in Atlanta had to do so at altitude in Columbia.

Dwellers at sea level are generally disadvantaged when competing at altitude. Some individuals are more affected than others and need to place greater attention on their preparation for such conditions. The physiological adaptations that occur as a result of a period of exposure to altitude may benefit subsequent performance at sea-level. This idea has prompted the use of training camps based at altitude. Hypobaric huts and normobaric hypoxic rooms where the proportion of oxygen in the air or its partial pressure can be manipulated have been developed to simulate altitude characteristics. Nevertheless, there is not a consensus among sports scientists as to whether there is a net benefit of training at altitude for sea-level performance.

PHYSIOLOGICAL BACKGROUND

The main physiological challenge caused by exercise at altitude is hypoxia. The air is less dense as ambient pressure decreases and, as there are fewer oxygen molecules in a given volume of air, less oxygen is inspired. The decrease in alveolar oxygen tension results in a lowered oxygen delivery by the red blood cells to the active tissues. Consequently, performances that rely on aerobic metabolism are adversely affected. The body does demonstrate some adaptive responses which compensate for the relative lack of oxygen in the air. These responses begin immediately on exposure to altitude but for some people the full response is not manifested until weeks or months there. Even with complete adaptation, the sea-level visitor to altitude is never as completely adjusted as the individual born and bred there. This ceiling is apparent in the case of endurance sports in particular.

The quest to reach ever greater heights than hitherto attained has been reflected in the attempts to climb the high peaks of the Himalayas, to achieve altitude records for hot-air ballooning and to parachute or hang-glide from new record heights. The difficulties encountered at great altitude have a rich history of documentation; the associated physical distress on the high mountains became known as mountain sickness. The problems are a result of hypoxia which prevails whenever atmospheric pressure drops subnormally, the decreases in ambient pressure being directly related to the heights reached. Symptoms usually appear within 24 hours and include nausea, headache, vomiting, and difficulties in breathing and sleeping. Onset may be sudden when ascent is rapid and there is a wide individual variability. Some people succumb at 2000 m, most are affected at 6500 m.

Normally the atmospheric pressure is 760 Torr (760 mmHg or 1 atm). As 20.93% of ambient air is oxygen, the partial pressure of oxygen in the air is 159 Torr. The important factor as far as breathing is concerned is the oxygen tension (PO_2) in the alveoli. Here the water vapour pressure is relatively constant at 47 Torr as is the CO_2 tension of 35–40 Torr. Consequently, the normal gradient for alveolar and venous PO_2 is 104 to 40 Torr which favours the transfer of oxygen through the pulmonary capillaries into the bloodstream. The gradient for CO_2 is in the reverse direction as PCO_2 in venous blood is normally 46 Torr, favouring elimination of CO_2 from the body via the lungs. With greater altitude the air becomes less dense and,

Table 4.1 Fall in alveolar PO_2 and % O_2 saturation of red blood cells with increasing altitude

Altitude [feet (m)]	Barometric Pressure (Torr)	PO_2 Tracheal Air (Torr)	% Arterial Saturation
0 (0)	760	149	97
10,000 (3200)	525	100	90
20,000 (6400)	350	63	70

though the percentage of oxygen in the air is unchanged, the tension falls due to the smaller number of oxygen molecules in a given volume of air. The result is an increased difficulty in getting oxygen into the blood. This process requires an increased ventilation rate to boost the alveolar oxygen tension, which is mainly achieved by a greater depth of breathing. This adjustment occurs immediately on exposure to hypoxia. The mechanisms involved are the peripheral chemoreceptors in the carotid and aortic bodies which respond to lowered arterial PO_2 and thus provide the drive to the respiratory centre in the medulla to stimulate an increase in ventilation. The stimulus is inevitably damped as a result of partial compensations brought about by effects of changes in arterial PCO_2 and in the pH of cerebrospinal fluid on the central chemoreceptors in the medulla.

The fall in arterial PCO_2 arises from the adaptive hyperventilatory response which causes excess CO_2 to be blown off from the blood passing through the lungs. Carbon dioxide is a weak acid in solution and its elimination leaves the blood more alkaline because of the excess bicarbonate ions; the condition is referred to as respiratory alkalosis. The base excess is slowly excreted by the kidneys over a few days, thereby returning the blood pH and its acid-base status towards normal. This means that the alkaline reserve is now reduced and so the blood has a poorer buffering capacity for coping with additional fixed acids entering it. Consequently, lactic acid diffusing from muscle into blood during exercise at altitude will be less easily neutralized and may cause an earlier decline in physical performance than would occur at sea-level. Meanwhile the buffering capacity of the muscle gradually improves in order to compensate.

The hypocapnia (low CO_2) has a vasoconstrictor effect on cerebral blood vessels although this effect is insufficient to offset the vasodilator stimulus for the cerebral resistance vessels provided by hypoxia. The vasoconstrictor response is attributed to an alkaline shift in the vessel wall which tends to protect the brain from alkalosis by retaining CO_2 by means of a decreased blood flow. The overall result, though, is a vasodilation and this net effect seems to be implicated in acute mountain sickness. The deterioration in mental functions, however, seems to be related to hydrolase reactions that impair the synthesis of an important neurotransmitter, dopamine.[1]

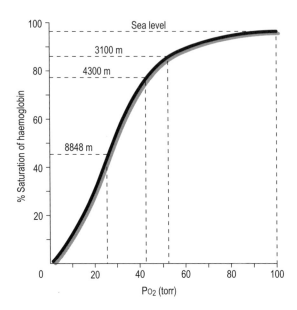

Figure 4.1 The standard oxygen dissociation curve of haemoglobin for a blood pH of 7.4 and body temperature of 37°C. The horizontal lines indicate % haemoglobin saturation of arterial blood at the different altitudes whilst the vertical lines indicate PO_2

Table 4.1 shows the drop in inspired or tracheal PO_2 with increases in altitude. Included also is the change in the carrying capacity of red blood cells shown as the percentage oxygen saturation. This change is because the oxygen dissociation curve of haemoglobin is affected by pressure, as shown in Figure 4.1. The blood leaving the pulmonary capillaries is normally 97% saturated with approximately 19 ml O_2 contained per 100 ml blood, the haemoglobin concentration being about 15 mg/dl. The curve is sigmoid in shape, being little affected for the first 1000-1500 m of altitude because of the flatness at the top but, as the pressure drops further to reach the steep part of the curve, the supply of oxygen to the body tissues is increasingly impaired. Loss of consciousness may be imminent when the saturation falls below 60%. The respiratory alkalosis of altitude serves to shift this curve to the left which assists in moving more oxygen into the blood. Though the circulatory system also shows acute responses including an increased cardiac output during exercise, mainly due to an increased heart rate, the maximal aerobic power inevitably declines. The impairment in aerobic power is usually manifest at about 1500 m in most individuals (and below that in athletes with a high $\dot{V}O_2$ max who may desaturate at high exercise intensities when performing at sea-level). A given work-rate, therefore, places a greater relative physiological strain on the individual at altitude so that aerobic performance is adversely affected.

EXTREME ALTITUDE

The earliest studies of the effects of altitude were concerned with balloonists. Competitive ballooning between European citizens was a matter of some prestige in the nineteenth century, British and French specialists notably vying with each other to attain the greater heights. Glaisher, a meteorologist at the Royal Observatory at Greenwich, ascended to an altitude estimated to be about 11 km in 1862.[2] He collapsed in the basket as a result of hypoxia and it was left to his companion to vent hydrogen from the balloon to allow it to descend. The companion had already lost the use of his hands as a result of the lack of oxygen and was forced to use his teeth to grip the cord that controlled the release valve, moving his head to release the required amount of gas. A more tragic fate befell the two colleagues of the famous scientist Tissandier in the French balloon Zenith a few years later. Their story illustrated dramatically the adverse effects of hypoxia on mental judgements. Tissandier[3] recounted that he realized his difficulty in breathing and the loss of use of his arms but felt happy that a height of 8 km was exceeded and that they were still rising. The balloon then drifted downwards for over a kilometre and he was aware that his colleagues were unconscious. Despite this occurrence, he released more ballast and ascended further once again to an estimated altitude of 8600 m. On returning to the ground both companions were found to have died, a fact that made national news headlines in France. At this time the oxygen supply systems were primitive and the gas was difficult to inhale, being bubbled through wash bottles to reduce the unpleasant smell coming from the oxygen containers.

The current oxygen supply systems are a considerable improvement on these versions and they enable great heights to be attained. Ross and Prather in the USA succeeded in flying a balloon over the Gulf of Mexico at a height of 34,668 m in 1961. Helium has replaced hydrogen as the gas of choice in many balloons and sojourners tend to aim for distance travelled at moderate or low heights rather than altitude reached. This makes the activity much safer than in its pioneering years when there was little real understanding of the physiological hazards involved. In recent years there have been many attempts to traverse the globe in hot-air balloons that have ended as dramatic failures. There have also been spectacular failures in launching of balloons for record attempts to high altitudes (about 40 km).

Mountaineering is the main sport that has provoked research into effects of hypoxia at extreme terrestrial altitudes. Provision of accessory oxygen was for many years considered to be essential if the earth's highest peaks in the Himalayas were to be climbed. Though scientists in the nineteenth century carried out experiments in low-pressure environmental chambers, it was not until the beginning of the twentieth century that the first high altitude research station was established. This was set up in 1907 by the Italian physiologist Mosso on one of the peaks of Monte Rosa in the Alps with financial support from Queen Margherita. In 1909 an Italian climber, the Duke of the Abruzzi, reached an altitude of 7500 m in the Karakorum Mountains without supplementary oxygen. In 1924 two British climbers,

Norton and Sommervell, exceeded 8500 m on the north side of Mount Everest, again without using accessory oxygen. Ten years later four climbers reached 8534 m on Everest without supplementary oxygen, though one repeatedly suffered from hallucinations.[4] In 1951 a British research team worked for three weeks in a tented laboratory at 5486 m and laid the foundations for planning the successful British Everest Expedition in 1953. Climbers who reached the summit of Everest (8850 m), Edmund Hillary and the sherpa Tensing Norgay, used an open circuit oxygen system but while at the top they were able to remove their breathing masks for 10 minutes.

The climbing of Everest seemed to break a psychological barrier for top-flight mountaineers who realised that the other high peaks of the Himalayas were all within physiological limits. The Himalayan mountains contain the world's seventeen highest peaks, all a challenge to mountaineers. Within three years of the first Everest conquest, the six highest peaks in the world had been climbed. The second highest mountain, K2 at 8611 m, and Cho Oyn (8200 m) were both climbed in 1954. Then the following year Kangchenjunga (8595 m) and Makalu (8470 m) were both conquered and Lhotse, the world's fourth highest peak, was first reached in 1956. The Japanese climber Junko Tabei in 1975 became the first woman to reach the summit of Everest. The Austrian climbers, Messner and Habeler, created new standards in 1978 when they reached the summit of Everest without supplementary oxygen. This spurred other expeditions to seek similar achievements and to tackle other high peaks without the support of oxygen equipment. Alternative goals now include the climbing of the highest peaks by hitherto unused routes, presenting a new type of challenge to the technical skills of the modern climber. After an already distinguished mountaineering career, the British climber Chris Bonington made his first climb to the summit of Everest in 1985 at the age of 50. A week later an American mountaineer, five years older than Bonington, performed the same feat. In 2000 Davo Karnicar made the first ski descent from the summit. A year later Nepalese student Temba Tsheri became the youngest person to reach the mountain top, followed a year later by Tomiyasu Ishikawa, the oldest at 65 years. These feats were again surpassed on the 50th anniversary of the first climbing of Everest when a 15-year-old Sherpa girl, Ming Kipa, and a 70-year-old male Japanese climber reached the summit in the same week (see Box 4.1). By the time the 50th anniversary of the first success was celebrated, over 1200 people had climbed to the summit and 150 had died in the attempt to do so. Indeed the intrinsic attraction of Everest to top climbers is exemplified by the fact that it is currently booked up by climbing expeditions for the next eight years.

There are now various research centres concerned with the study of high altitude physiology. The most notable are those in the Andes, in Colorado and in the Alps. There have also been meritorious studies on the high mountains conducted in temporary installations. A British expedition to the Himalayas in 1960-61 set up a prefabricated hut at an altitude of 5800 m (380 Torr pressure) to base a physiological research team there for five months of the winter. Extensive studies were made on the physiological processes of

Box 4.1 Chronology of notable achievements in climbing Mount Everest

1865	The mountain is named Everest after the British Surveyor General
1921	George Mallory and Guy Bullock reach North Col at 7000 m
1924	Ill-fated attempt by Mallory and Irvine to reach the top
	Norton and Sommervall reach 8500 m without accessory oxygen
1953	Edmund Hillary and Tensing Norgay reach the summit
1960	Chinese-Tibetan group claim to reach the top via North Col and North East ridge
1975	Junko Tabei, Japan, becomes the first woman to the summit
1978	Reinhold Messner and Peter Habeler complete climb without supplementary oxygen
1979	First solo ascent by Messner
1998	Tom Whitaker becomes first amputee to reach the summit
2002	Apa Sherpa (Nepal) climbs Everest for the 12th time
2003	Yuichiro Miura (Japan) is first 70-year old to climb the mountain.
	Ming Kipa (Nepal) at 15 is youngest climber to reach the top
	Fastest climb from Base Camp to top, 10 h 55 min

adaptation to altitude[5] and the researchers subsequently made measurements of $\dot{V}O_{2\,max}$ during cycle ergometry at an altitude of 7440 m (300 Torr).

One of the most impressive research projects using mobile laboratories at extreme altitude was the American Medical Research Expedition to Everest in 1981.[6] The group consisted of climbers and scientists along with six individuals who were scientists-cum-climbers with a high level of fitness. Research laboratories were set up at 5400 m (400 Torr), 6300 m (351 Torr) and 8050 m (283 Torr) while alveolar gas, pulmonary ventilation and ECG were studied on the summit.[7,8]

Results confirmed that the peak of Everest is just within the limits of human tolerance. They showed that it was possible for two well-acclimatized subjects to reach an oxygen uptake in excess of 1 l/min when the inspired PO_2 was 43 Torr as it is on the summit. The very low PCO_2 levels caused by extreme hyperventilation help to maintain the alveolar PO_2 despite a greatly reduced inspired value. Barometric pressure measured on the summit (253 Torr) was not as low as the 236 Torr predicted using the International Civil Aviation Organisation's Standard Atmosphere regression line. Indeed, the physiological reserve at this height is so marginal that day-to-day variations

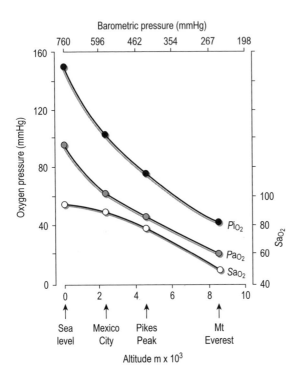

Figure 4.2 Changes in barometric pressure, inspired partial pressure of oxygen (PO$_2$), alveolar oxygen tension (PO$_2$) and oxyhaemoglobin saturation at altitude

in pressure can mean the difference between success and failure in climbing assaults on the summit (see Figure 4.2).

HIGH ALTITUDES

Tolerance to high altitudes may well be beyond the capacity of many unacclimatized individuals, especially if the level of fitness is not impressive. Indeed, evidence suggests that a height of 5900 m (18,000 feet) is about the limit of permanent human habitation, the oxygen saturation at this altitude being lowered to nearly 70%. The highest permanent human settlement is in the Andes (5500 m) and it seems that above this altitude acclimatization is replaced by a steady deterioration. Chilean mineworkers complain of loss of sleep and appetite when sleeping 300 m above this level, where discomfort is also encountered by seasonal mountaineers. Prolonged stops lead to the so-called 'high altitude deterioration'; factors involved are water loss and heat loss in vigorous hyperventilation of dry air, sweating induced by solar radiation reflected from snow on the mountains, muscle atrophy and loss of strength, poor nutritional status, loss of appetite, mental stress, lack of sleep and illness.

Table 4.2 Altitude illnesses[29]

Acute Hypoxia	Mental impairment and usual collapse after rapid exposure above 5500m (18,000 feet).
Acute Mountain Sickness	Headache, nausea, vomiting, sleep disturbance, dyspnoea at above 2100-2500 m (7000-8000 feet): it is common and self limited.
High Altitude Pulmonary Oedema	Dyspnoea, cough, weakness, headache, stupor and rarely death. 2750-3050 m and above (9000-10,000 feet): it requires rapid descent or early treatment.
High Altitude Cerebral Oedema	Severe headache, hallucinations, ataxia, weakness, impaired thinking, stupor or death. Above 3050-3550 m (10,000-12,000 feet); Uncommon. Descent is mandatory.
Subacute and Chronic Mountain Sickness	Failure to recover from acute mountain sickness may necessitate descent. Dyspnoea, fatigue, plethora and heart failure may develop after years of asymptomatic residence at altitude.
Chronic conditions worsened by altitude	Sickle trait, chronic cardiac or pulmonary disease
High Altitude Deterioration	Long periods spent above 5500 m (18,000 feet): cause insomnia, fatigue, weight loss and general deterioration. Deterioration is more rapid at higher altitudes

Sojourners are vulnerable to various forms of altitude sicknesses at moderately high altitudes, a detailed list of these and their symptoms being contained in Table 4.2. Many of the illnesses stem from the biological repercussions of the respiratory alkalosis induced by hyperventilation and the alteration in blood flow to the brain provoked by hypoxia. It is clear that sojourns above about 5000 m need to be planned so that target climbs are completed within a restricted period of time.

The muscle-wasting effects of prolonged stays at medium to high altitude have been linked with suppression of appetite and the consequent reduction in energy intake. Climbers find that food is less appetising with increased altitude and need to be encouraged to continue to eat. The depression of appetite has been associated with increased output of neuropeptides within the gut. There have been suggestions that hyperphagic effects of antioxidant supplementation at high altitude can help to raise self-chosen energy intake, as well as reduce the severity of acute mountain sickness.[10]

Sports activities at this level of hypobaric stress are mainly limited to mountaineering, skiing and some athletic competitions on land, and aerial sports such as gliding and parachuting. The highest cities in which important international games are held include Bogota in Columbia and La Paz in Bolivia. Four of the top Bolivian football clubs play at an altitude above 3000 m and one of its clubs, El Alto, plays its home matches above 4000 m. Soccer teams visiting these venues from sea-level nations suffer distress if prior acclimatization has been ignored beforehand. Columbia has hosted the world swimming championships and Bolivia the Copa America soccer championships in 1997. A mountain race up to about 4000 m on Mount Fako, Cameroun in West Africa, is now an annual competitive event. The risks associated with unfit sedentary individuals going to high altitude resorts for recreational skiing should be recognized and their activity programmes modified accordingly. Even greater caution should be taken with middle-aged people flying to the high resorts for trekking holidays, as many tour operators show a total disregard for the physiological strain involved.

MODERATE ALTITUDES

It is now common for major international competitions to be held at moderate altitudes between 1500 m and 2500 m. Earliest experience of major games at the altitudes were international rugby and athletics meetings in Johannesberg, South Africa (1800 m) and the 1955 Pan American Games in Mexico (2280 m). Locating the 1968 Olympic Games and the 1970 and 1986 soccer World Cup competitions in Mexico precipitated a flurry of research projects into the physiological effects of altitude. Projects were conducted in environmental chambers based at ground level, or involved transport of sea-level dwellers to research laboratories or field conditions at about 2300 m. A common observation was a deterioration in $\dot{V}O_{2\,max}$ of 14%, though a four-week stay reduced this drop to 9%.[9] It is calculated that $\dot{V}O_{2\,max}$ is reduced by 2-3% for every 250 m ascent between 1500 m and 6100 m.[10] The experiments that took athletes higher than Mexico City but provided them with pure oxygen to breathe, showed clearly that cardiac output was affected through a reduction in either the pumping power of the myocardium or the venous return of blood to the heart. Another problem foreseen before the 1968 Olympic Games was the effect that the increased breathing rate could have on rhythmic events such as swimming and rowing where the breathing frequency is normally synchronized with the stroke rate. It seemed essential that sea-level dwellers should acclimatize to altitude before competing seriously there.

The predictions of the scientists were borne out in the performances at the Olympic Games in Mexico City, the long distance races being mostly affected.

All medalists in running events of 800 m distance or longer were either living at altitude or had experienced prolonged spells there for training purposes. The reduced air density enhanced performance in the sprint events, creating less resistance to movement. Indeed the phenomenal performances by Bob Beamon in the long jump and Lee Evans in the 400 m were still unsurpassed four Olympiads later. Subsequently many other notable sprinting feats have been accomplished at altitude. In the throwing events, javelin and discus throwing depend on the aerodynamic properties of the missiles and so performance is not necessarily enhanced by the thinner air.

Ideally, preparation for endurance performance at altitude requires a period of acclimatization. This advice is extended to psychomotor performance that is also affected by hypoxia. As many altitude natives are noted to perform well at sea-level – Colombian runners and cyclists, runners from the highlands of Kenya and Ethiopia, for example – the reasoning amongst practitioners is that altitude acclimatization can be used to assist subsequent performance at sea-level.

The use of altitude training needs to be systematized, not only in terms of frequency and duration of sojourns, level of altitude and intensity of training programmes but also in the timing of the return to sea-level. Over the last three decades the use of altitude training has been incorporated into the annual calendar of elite athletes in a variety of sports. Others use environmental chambers or 'hypoxic huts' to gain the benefits of physiological adaptation. The individual nature of responses to altitude and the compounding of physiological factors with the so-called 'training camp effect' make it difficult for scientists to present simple answers. In the environment of the training camp, athletes tend to benefit from the focus on physical preparation and the availability of a range of supportive expertise. It is correctly felt by practitioners that astute use of altitude training can enhance endurance performance potential for sea-level contests. Sports scientists, however, try to weigh the positive benefits of the adaptations that take place against those that would adversely affect the performance of vigorous exercise.

EFFECTS OF MODERATE ALTITUDE ON EXERCISE PERFORMANCE

The maximal aerobic power ($\dot{V}O_{2\,max}$) is reduced by about 15% at an altitude of 2.3 km. (It is estimated that $\dot{V}O_{2\,max}$ declines by about 1-2% for every 100 m above 1.5 km.) After 3-4 weeks at altitude, a portion of this impairment is recovered but the $\dot{V}O_{2\,max}$ remains below sea-level values. For example, the 15% initial drop in $\dot{V}O_{2\,max}$ at an altitude of 2.3 km is reversed to 9% of the sea-level value within 4 weeks. These average values mask a wide variation between individuals. There is also a reduction in the maximal heart rate that is reached at altitude.

The fall in maximal aerobic power as a consequence of the reduction in ambient air pressure means that a fixed exercise challenge imposes a greater physiological stress on the athlete. Consequently higher blood lactate values

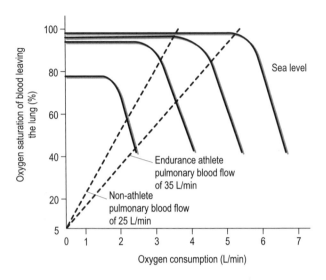

Figure 4.3 Comparison of the alveolar-arterial oxygen difference between untrained individuals and endurance trained athletes at maximal exercise. After Levine B. Training and exercise at high altitudes[19]

are observed compared with the same work-rate at sea-level and the increase corresponds to the decrease in $\dot{V}O_{2\,max}$. This decline has implications for games players in particular, since longer periods than normal are required to clear the lactate that is produced and accumulates in the bloodstream. Alongside the increased relative physiological stress is a rise in the perceived exertion. A consequence is that the training intensity that can be tolerated is lower than at sea-level.

Trained individuals experience greater reductions in $\dot{V}O_{2\,max}$ whilst exercising in acute hypoxic conditions than untrained subjects.[11] This finding is consistent with the hypothesis that trained subjects experience greater pulmonary diffusion limitations to $\dot{V}O_{2\,max}$ than untrained subjects during maximal exercise. Individuals who are aerobically well trained (but not necessarily acclimatized) generally have an immediate decrease in $\dot{V}O_{2\,max}$ at an inspired PO_2 of about 130 mmHg, corresponding to an altitude of 600-900 m above sea-level. In contrast, sedentary individuals are unaffected up to at least 1200 m.[12] Above this altitude the oxygen-haemoglobin (O_2-Hb) saturation curve starts to decline steeply and affects the oxygen transport system. Oxygen moves between the alveoli in the lungs and the arterial blood by dissolving and diffusing through the alveolar membranes and interstitial spaces. Diffusion limitation across the pulmonary capillaries may occur at lower altitudes in the endurance athlete compared to the untrained individual, largely because in the former, improvements in cardiac output with training are not matched by changes in diffusion capacity (see Figure 4.3).

The decline in $\dot{V}O_{2\,max}$ is mirrored in a decrease in distance running performance. The experimental work undertaken at Mexico City in the year

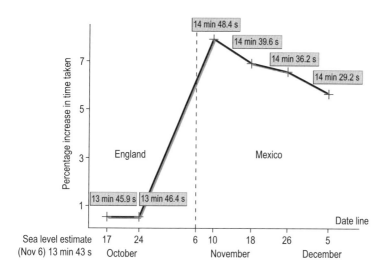

Figure 4.4 Mean performance of six British athletes in 3-mile time trials before and during a one-month stay at an altitude of 2300 m in 1967 (reproduced with permission of the British Olympic Association)

prior to the 1968 Olympics demonstrated a deterioration in time to run three miles.[9] Sea-level performance (13 min 46 s) deteriorated at altitude by 62 s but improved over the next 4 weeks at altitude by 19 s on average (see Figure 4.4).

The reduction in air density at altitude means that performance may be improved at events where air resistance is a limiting factor. This applies to throwing events, jumping and sprinting. It is notable that world records at the Mexico City Olympics were set in track events at all distances up to and including 800 m. The contribution of the reduced air density (and wind assistance) to the world record of Bob Beamon in the long jump was calculated to be 0.31 m.[13] The main factor was the increased run-up speed attainable under these favourable conditions.

Altitude can present difficulties to games players over and above the physiological challenges. One problem is that the ball travels more easily through the thinner air. This can cause difficulty in both shooting and clearing the ball by long kicks out of defence. The goalkeeper in soccer may also be more easily deceived by shots at goal, owing to the faster ball flight. Games players need to consider the altered ball behaviour when either running or chasing the ball. Finally, some concessions in game tactics may need to be made for players particularly vulnerable to altitude deterioration.

ACUTE ADAPTATIONS

The reduction in partial pressure of oxygen in the inspired air is the source of the unique stress on sports performers at altitude. As mentioned earlier, the immediate physiological adjustment to altitude exposure is an increase in minute ventilation to boost the partial oxygen tension (PO_2) in the pulmonary alveoli. This helps in part to offset the fall in oxygen saturation that follows the reduction in alveolar PO_2.

The drop in O_2 saturation may not lead to a decline in the oxygen transport system until an altitude of about 1200 m is reached, although this value is subject to individual differences (in particular the level of aerobic fitness). This non-linear response is because of the sigmoid shape of the O_2-Hb saturation curve. Oxygen desaturation may occur at high exercise intensities at lower altitudes in well-trained endurance athletes. These may therefore experience greater deterioration in their aerobic performance when exercising at altitude than do untrained individuals.

The respiratory compensation response to hypoxia leads to a rise in blood pH as a result of CO_2 being lost via hyperventilation. As CO_2 in solution is a weak acid, the blood is more alkaline than normal because of the excess of bicarbonate ions. The kidneys respond by excreting bicarbonate over several days which helps to restore blood pH towards normal. The alkaline reserve is temporarily decreased by this process and so, until the buffering capacity increases with acclimatisation, the blood has a poorer capability for tolerating entry of additional acids (such as lactic acid) into it. Lactic acid diffusing from active muscles into the blood during exercise at altitude will not be neutralized as easily as normal. High intensity performance declines earlier than at sea-level as a result, and the intensity of aerobic training needs to be lowered for training sessions to be sustained.

Muscle buffering capacity increases, partially compensating for the reduction in blood alkaline reserve. The low oxygen tension does not significantly affect the uptake of oxygen by the red blood cells until the oxygen pressure declines to a certain point. However, with adaptation to altitude the critical oxygen pressure falls. This results from increased production of 2,3-bisphosphoglycerate (BPG) by the red blood cells, and is beneficial in that it aids the unloading of oxygen from the red cells at the tissues. The oxygen-carrying capacity of the blood is enhanced by an increase in the number of red blood cells.

Within a few days of reaching an altitude location, a rise in haemoglobin concentration is apparent, but this initial increase in haemoglobin is a result of haemoconcentration owing to a drop in plasma volume. Nevertheless, there is a gradual true increase in haemoglobin which is mediated by stimulation of the bone marrow to produce more red blood cells by erythropoiesis. The increased production of red blood cells requires that the body's iron stores are adequate and may indeed mean supplementation of iron intake prior to and during the stay at altitude. A check that serum ferritin stores are adequate is an important screening procedure to ensure that the athlete can benefit from exposure to altitude.

The bone marrow increases its iron uptake to form haemoglobin after about 48 hours at altitude. If the individual remains at high altitude, it takes 2-3 weeks to secure a true increase in total body haemoglobin and the red cell count continues to increase for one year or more but does not attain the values observed in high-altitude natives. As the haemoglobin concentration increases, there is an associated rise in the haematocrit. The red cell mass is still increasing after 36 weeks, approaching values seen in residents at high altitude.

On first exposure to altitude there is an increase in heart rate response to submaximal exercise. Successful adaptation to altitude results in a reduction in the heart rate response to a near normal level.

The endocrine system is also sensitive to altitude hypoxia and responds in a number of ways. Stimulation of the adrenal cortex by secretion of ACTH from the pituitary gland represents part of a generalized stress reaction. After some weeks at altitude up to 6300 m, cortisol levels return to their baseline sea-level values. Exercise stimulates release of renin and aldosterone, the latter being the most important hormone in regulating sodium concentrations by its effect on the kidneys. Acute exposure to altitude causes a drop in resting aldosterone but during exercise the response of aldosterone to a rise in renin is blunted. Higher aldosterone levels and therefore greater sodium retention are found on arrival at altitude in subjects who suffer acute mountain sickness compared to those who turn out to be resistant to it.[14] Sodium diuresis is promoted by atrial natriuretic peptide and this hormone plays a role in maintaining plasma volume when sodium concentration increases. Antidiuretic hormone does not change at altitude, at least in those free of acute mountain sickness, but becomes elevated in individuals with pulmonary oedema or who become sick and vomit.

METABOLIC ADAPTATIONS

At extreme altitudes, increases in alveolar ventilation and decreases in mixed venous oxygen content are primarily responsible for maintaining exercise capacity despite severe hypoxia. The mechanisms that assist performance at sea-level following exposure to moderate altitude may be different. The major adaptation in this case may be the increases in haemoglobin and haematocrit consequent to the stimulation of erythropoiesis.[15] The changes in blood may be complemented by changes at tissue level including increased myoglobin, capillary density and mitochondrial activities.

Anaerobic capacity also may be positively affected by short stays at altitude.[16] Changes include alterations in lactate dehydrogenase isoform pattern and in muscle buffer capacity. Such changes persist for two weeks on return to sea-level: changes in muscle buffer capacity were correlated with improved performance time in cross-country skiers following a period of altitude training. Saltin[17] considered that improved performances in activities taxing aerobic and anaerobic systems may be attributable to an improved anaerobic capacity. This suggestion is supported by studies at cellular level where adaptation to hypoxia is brought about by means of a transcriptional factor, hypoxia-inducible factor 1 (HIF-1). Activation of HIF-1 is necessary for the induction of several genes including those encoding for erythropoietin, vascular endothelial growth factor, GLUT-1 transporter (which helps in the movement of glucose across the cell membrane) and several glycolytic enzymes.[18] Improvements in mRNA concentrations for phosphofructokinase after training at altitude would also constitute an increased capability for anaerobic performance.

Adaptations to altitude may occur at any of the steps in the oxygen cascade between the lungs and the muscle cells. Ventilatory and circulatory adaptations are complemented by increased peripheral uptake of oxygen by the active muscles. This improvement could be due to increased mitochondrial activities, capillarization and tissue myoglobin as well as increased concentrations of 2,3-BPG.[19]

Acclimatization may improve both oxygen delivery and extraction, oxygen carrying capacity being enhanced by the increased red cell mass, and unloading at tissue level being increased by the increase in 2,3-BPG. Additionally, substrate utilization is enhanced by mobilization of free fatty acids and increased use of blood glucose, thereby saving muscle glycogen.[20]

The success of East African middle-distance and long-distance runners in major competitions has led to the belief that their excellent performances are linked to their living in natural highlands. Whilst the Kenyan runners tend to have $\dot{V}O_{2\,max}$ values of 82 ml/kg/min, and a blunted ammonia response to exercise compared to Europeans,[21] the difference between East African and European teenagers is small. This observation led Saltin[17] to the conclusion that the success of the Kenyan athletes is attributable more to strenuous training than to hypoxia, and to the large pool of well-conditioned youngsters in the country.

The opportunity to take advantage of altitude training depends either on an accident of birth or the financial support available to the sea-level dweller. Even then, exposure to altitude demands careful attention to physiological detail so that adverse effects (such as acute mountain sickness) are avoided and the training stimulus is carefully matched to the prevailing capability of the individual.

ALTITUDE TRAINING CAMPS

Altitude training to enhance subsequent performance capability at sea-level is now widely used by sea-level natives in a range of sports. Such a manoeuvre is legal and has spawned the development of training camps based at altitude resorts.

The use of altitude training camps for enhancement of sea-level performances received renewed interest in the 1990s amongst many sports coaches. Middle-distance and long-distance runners from the UK had used a range of altitude locations including Albuquerque (1500 m) and Mexico City (2280 m). The difference in these two exposures was reflected in a significant increase in haemoglobin and haematocrit concentration in Mexico but no change after Albuquerque. It seemed that an altitude in excess of 2000 m and up to 2500 m, when the reduction in ambient pressure takes the oxygen-saturation curve of haemoglobin into a steep decline, is needed to induce an appreciable adaptive effect on red cell mass.

In rowers, particular attention has been given to reducing the training load on early exposure in order to avoid acute mountain sickness. Later, individuals have been carefully programmed with increased training loads whilst metabolic responses were regularly recorded.[22] The training programme takes into account the competitive schedule following return to sea-level. There is not a complete consensus on the optimal timing of this return to sea-level before participation in major competition but most practitioners believe performance peaks just 15 days after descent from altitude.

Ingjer and Myhre[23] studied Swedish skiers for a similar three-week period at 1.9 km with a subsequent long-term follow up. A strict liquid intake regimen was effective in reducing the fall in plasma volume associated with dehydration at altitude. The blood lactate response to a sub-maximal exercise test was lowered immediately on return to sea-level, illustrating a beneficial response. This decrease was correlated with the increase in haemoglobin and haematocrit that occurred at altitude. It seems that the individuals who benefit most from altitude training are those with the greatest room for elevating oxygen-carrying capacity. The level of altitude seemingly influences the stimulatory effect of erythropoietin. At about 1900 m the rise in serum erythropoietin is apparent after approximately one week at altitude, and this may be associated with increased oxygenation of the tissues owing to 2,3-BPG. The true rise in haemoglobin averages approximately 1% each week, at least at altitudes between 1.8 and 3 km.[24]

It is estimated that optimal haematological adaptations to altitude take around 80 days to accrue. This schedule may be accelerated by periodic visits to higher altitude (up to 3 km) but not training there. The inability to tolerate high training loads at altitude may lead to a drop in aerobic fitness which offsets the positive effects of the altitude sojourn. If the oxygen saturation declines to a level where the exercise intensity falls off below that required to maintain current fitness, then performance will suffer. The answer may be a combination of living at altitude for a sustained period but frequently returning to near sea-level (locally if possible) for strenuous exercise training. The best combination seems to be to live at about 2.8 km but train at below 2 km, represented by the 'live high, train low' philosophy.[19]

Upon return to sea-level it will take a few days for the acid-base status to be re-established. Hypoxia no longer stimulates erythropoiesis and the elevated red cell count slowly comes down. The decreased affinity of red blood cells for oxygen, which facilitated its unloading to the active tissues by means of the activity of 2,3-BPG, is soon lost on return to sea-level. Any exploitation of the haematological adaptation must be carefully timed to occur before the red blood cell count returns to normality: this process may take up to six weeks. Otherwise, repeated sojourns to altitude are needed to maintain benefits.

SIMULATED ALTITUDE

Hypoxic huts (where the ambient O_2 pressure is reduced by increasing the nitrogen content of the air) and hypobaric chambers provide opportunities for athletes to spend time in hypoxic conditions in attempts to induce the physiological adjustments associated with altitude exposure. These facilities may be used for training purposes or can be used as temporary residence. The hypoxic stimulus is accentuated by sleeping in the hut, as the alveolar PO_2 drops during sleep.

Terrados et al.[25] demonstrated that continuous exercise of 60-90 minutes, performed four or five times each week at a simulated altitude of 2300 m, showed good results in three to four weeks. Similar effects were observed by means of an intermittent exercise protocol of 45-60 minutes. Later, Hendriksen and Meeuwsen[26] showed in a cross-over study that an intermittent exercise regimen improved both anaerobic power and maximal aerobic performance more when completed in hypobaric hypoxia compared to normal sea-level conditions. The results provide support for the use of simulated altitude as a training environment, although not all studies have been so conclusive. Enhanced effects may depend on the altitude simulated, the dimensions of the training programme and the initial fitness levels of the subjects.

Normobaric hypoxic rooms have become commercially available and purport to augment normal training effects (see Figure 4.5). Savourey et al.[27] compared responses to hypobaric hypoxia and normobaric hypoxia in order to establish whether the latter represented a true physiological simulation of altitude. Subjects were exposed for 40 minutes to a partial oxygen pressure of 120 kPa, equivalent to being at an altitude of 4500 m. Under hypobaric hypoxia the subjects displayed a greater breathing frequency and a lowered tidal volume suggestive of an increased dead space ventilation. Such a change would explain the lower blood alkalosis and a lowered oxygen arterial saturation evident in the hypobaric hypoxic trial. The increased dead space ventilation was attributed to the reduction in barometric pressure leading the authors to conclude that there were specific physiological responses to various levels of decrease in ambient pressure.

The effects of training are attributable to the relative exercise intensity experienced by the athlete. Since maximal oxygen is reduced in hypoxic environments, a given submaximal work-rate induces a greater relative physiological strain as reflected in an elevation in heart rate and blood lactate. This increase in relative intensity means that use of simulated altitude could be justified for strategic purposes, such as maintaining aerobic fitness in athletes during their rehabilitation from injury.

Portable altitude simulators in which the inspired O_2 tension is reduced have been designed for use as a back-pack whilst training. They are effective in altering the ventilatory response to exercise but may not induce any further adaptive benefit.[28] They may have psychological benefits by exposing athletes to the experience of hypoxia prior to visiting altitude resorts.

The hypoxic tent represents yet another means of attempting to replicate the altitude environment whilst remaining at sea-level. The device allows the athlete to sleep in hypoxic conditions whilst training during the day as normal. Air with a reduced oxygen content is pumped into the space

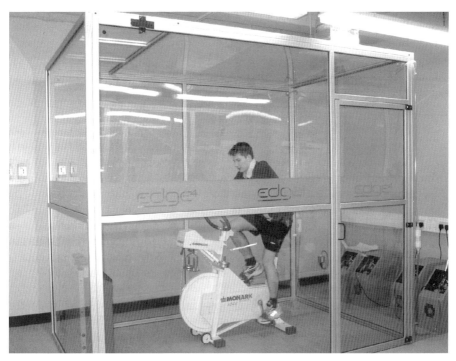

Figure 4.5 Athlete in a normobaric hypoxic exercise room at the Research Institute for Sport and Exercise Sciences at Liverpool John Moores University

contained in a canopy over the individual's bed, thereby reducing the partial pressure of the inspired oxygen. Such tents have the advantage of being transportable and have been taken on tours by some athletes. Sleep apnoea may be induced if the oxygen content within the tent falls below projected levels, for example if used without modification of the air breathed to take account of the prevailing altitude. Its physiological benefits and the psychological effects of sleeping in a restricted environment have not been adequately explored.

NON-RESPONDERS TO ALTITUDE TRAINING

There is a large variability in the effectiveness of altitude training for performance at sea-level. Some headway has been made in identifying the reasons why some athletes may acquire little or no benefit or why, for some individuals, altitude exposure may have a negative effect. It is essential that iron stores are sufficient if the athlete is to be able to realize the increase in red cell mass consequent to the increased production of erythropoietin. The increase in red cell mass is an essential component of any improvement in $\dot{V}O_{2\,max}$ due to altitude training. Athletes, particularly female athletes, may have low ferritin stores due to loss of blood during menses and, as a consequence, be unable to sustain the physiological requirements for red blood cell production. Athletes with low iron stores need supplementation and attention to diet three weeks or more prior to going to altitude.

Illness is a contraindication for going to an altitude training camp. An increased cytokine release associated with viral infections inhibits erythropoietin production as the bone marrow is stimulated instead to increase white blood cells. Individuals with infections will therefore be unable to exploit the hypoxic stimulus.

Similarly, injured athletes have increased inhibitory response to cytokines which means that erythropoietin is not stimulated. Furthermore, the sojourn to altitude may mean an inability to access medical treatment which is a priority when injured. For management of games teams, leaving an injured player out of the training camp squad may constitute a difficult decision to be balanced by possible effects on team morale.

It is important that athletes at altitude are adequately nourished. In particular, attention should be paid to the carbohydrate content of the diet in order to ensure glycogen stores are not reduced. With acclimatization there is a greater reliance on blood glucose and an increased use of fat as an energy source in order to spare muscle glycogen.

Finally, there is little point in taking unfit individuals to altitude for training purposes. Altitude training is not a substitute for training at sea-level with a well-planned regimen but rather in certain circumstances represents a method for honing fitness levels. The main reason for excluding unfit individuals is that they will be unable to exercise at an intensity to benefit from altitude and are better advised to train at sea-level where a higher absolute work-rate can be sustained.

OVERVIEW

The mountains have an alluring appeal to human adventurers that transcends understanding. The world's highest peaks pose extreme physiological challenges to mountaineers. The climber encounters hypoxia, cold and windy conditions as well as risks of avalanches and accidents. The prospects of suffering 'snow blindness' or succumbing to mountain sickness are added hazards. Scaling the high mountains is only possible when meticulous planning is combined with physiological preparation and favourable weather conditions. At moderate altitudes there are many who will struggle to cope with hypoxia and may experience so-called 'acute mountain sickness'. Even at lower altitudes the possibility of experiencing hypothermia is a real one, particularly when there is a rapid change in the balance between heat production and heat loss. Whilst the hypoxic environment is hostile for human habitation, there are physiological adjustments that allow the individual to cope. These adaptations have acute and more long-term phases, and have been exploited by elite athletes in preparing at altitude camps for competition at sea-level. Nevertheless, there is no mechanistic formula for successful use of altitude training and it should be seen as a supplement to, rather than a substitute for, a normal individualized programme.

References

1. Lassen NW. The brain, cerebral blood flow. In: Hypoxia: man at altitude. Sutton JR, Jones NL, Houston CS (eds). New York: Thieme Stratton, 1982

2. Glaisher J. Travels in the air. Philadelphia: Lippincott, 1871

3. Tissandier O. Le voyage a grande hauteur du ballon le Zenith. Nature Paris 1875; 3:337- 344

4. Ward M. Mountain medicine. London: Crosby Lockwood Staples, 1975

5. Pugh LGCE. Physiological and medical aspects of the Himalayan scientific and mountaineering expedition. BMJ 1962; 2:621-627

6. West JB, Lahiai S, Maret KH et al. Barometric pressures at extreme altitudes on Mount Everest: physiological significance. J Appl Physiol 1983; 54:1188-1194

7. West JB, Boyer SJ, Graber DJ et al. Maximal exercise at extreme altitudes on Mount Everest. J Appl Physiol, Respiration, Environ Exerc Physiol, 1983; 55:688-698

8. West JB, Hackett PH, Maret KH et al. Pulmonary gas exchange on the summit of Mount Everest. J Appl Physiol, Respiration, Environ Exerc Physiol, 1983; 55:678-687

9. Pugh LGCE. Athletes at altitude. J Physiol 1967; 192:619-646

10. Kollias J, Buskirk ER. Exercise at altitude. In: Science and medicine of exercise and sport. 2nd ed. Johnson WR, Buskirk ER (eds). New York: Harper and Row, 1974

11. Martin D, O'Kroy J. Effects of acute hypoxia on the $\dot{V}O_2$ max of trained and untrained subjects. J Sports Sci 1993; 11:37-42

12. Terrados N, Mizuno M, Anderson H. Reduction in maximal oxygen uptake at low altitudes: role of training status and lung function. Clin Physiol 1995; 5 (Suppl 3):75- 79

13. Ward-Smith AJ. Altitude and wind effects on long jump performance with particular reference to the world record established by Bob Beamon. J Sports Sci 1986; 4:89-99

14. Milledge JS. Altitude. In: Oxford textbook of sports medicine. 2nd ed. Harries M, Williams C, Stanish WD et al (eds). Oxford: Oxford Medical Publications, 1998:255-269

15. Levine BD, Stray-Gunderson J. A practical approach to altitude training: where to live and train for optimal performance enhancement. Int J Sports Med 1992; 13:S209-S212

16. Svedenhag J, Saltin B, Johansson C et al. Aerobic and anaerobic exercise capacities of elite middle-distance runners after two weeks of training at moderate altitude. Scand J Med Sci Sports 1991; 1:205-214

17. Saltin B. Exercise and the environment: focus on altitude. Res Quart Exerc Sport 1996; 67 (Suppl 3):1-10

18. Wenger RH, Gassmann M. Oxygen(es) and the hypoxia inducible factor - 1. Biol Chem 1997; 378:609-616

19. Levine B. Training and exercise at high altitudes. In: Atkinson G, Reilly T (eds). Sport, leisure and ergonomics III. London: E and FN Spon, 1995:74-92

20. Brooks G, Butterfield GA, Wolfe RR et al. Increased dependence on blood glucose after acclimatisation to 4300 m. J Appl Physiol 1991; 70:919-927

21. Saltin B, Larsen H, Terrados N. Aerobic exercise capacity at sea-level and at altitude in Kenyan boys, junior and senior runners compared with Scandinavian runners. Scan J Med Sci Sports 1995; 5:209-221

22. Grobler J, Faulmann L. The British experience. BOA Technical News 1993; 1(5):3-5

23. Ingjer F, Myhre K. Physiological effects of altitude training in young elite male cross-country skiers. J Sports Sci 1992; 10:45-63

24. Berglund B. High altitude training aspects of haematological adaptation. Sports Med 1992; 14:289-303

25. Terrados N, Melichna J, Sylven C et al. Effects of training and simulated altitude on performance and muscle metabolic capacity in competitive road cyclists. Eur J Appl Physiol 1988; 57:203-209

26. Hendriksen IJM, Meeuwsen T. The effect of intermittent training in hypobaric hypoxia on sea-level exercise: a cross-over study in humans. Europ J Appl Physiol 2003; 56:831-838
27. Savourey G, Launay JC, Besnard Y et al. Normo- and hypobaric hypoxia: are there physiological differences? Europ J Appl Physiol 2003; 89:122-126
28. Clucas N, Reilly T, McLean P. A portable simulator of altitude stress. In: Brown ID, Goldsmith R, Coombes K et al (eds). Proceedings of Ninth International Ergonomics Association Conference. London: Taylor & Francis, 1985:535-537
29. Houston CS. Oxygen lack at high altitude: a mountaineering problem. In: Hypoxia: man at altitude. Sutton JR, Jones NL, Houston CS (eds). New York: Thieme Stratton, 1982:156-157

Chapter 5

Underwater sports

CHAPTER CONTENTS

Introduction 73
Underwater stress 74
Skin diving 75
Scuba diving 79
Consequences of working under water
    80

Decompression 83
Cave diving 85
Hyperbaric exercise 86
Fitness for diving 87
Overview 87

INTRODUCTION

The underwater environment can be attractive for viewing its habitat and exploring its reefs or its submerged wrecks. Its allure is reflected in recreational activities such as caving, explorations, sports diving and so on. Research in underwater medicine has contributed to the understanding of how the human reacts in the event of increases in pressure underwater and exposure to cold water. This research has been supplemented by studies in naval research laboratories concerned with survival in hyperbaric environments and in oil companies concerned with oil exploration. In each case, technology has evolved so that the human can tolerate these inhospitable conditions and cope with their extreme dangers.

Increasingly, recreational divers are prepared to adopt technological developments from naval and commercial divers. The sports diver, caver, underwater photographer or spear fisherman progresses only to moderate depths compared to the professional diver. Nevertheless, a clear understanding of the relevant physical laws is important since the price of misinterpreting what is happening and adopting inappropriate remedial action can be death. Appreciation of fundamental physical laws forms the basis for this understanding.

The main physical stress on the body under water is due to the increased ambient pressure exerting a squeeze upon it. For roughly every 10 m descent (10.03 m sea water or 10.33 m fresh water), the external pressure increases by an equivalent of the atmospheric pressure (1 atm or 760 Torr) so that at a depth of 50 m the external pressure on the body is 6 atm. The main physiological challenge is presented by the need to breathe, since the time sustainable underwater without breathing oxygen is limited.

The tissues of the body are incompressible as a result of which their volume does not change, even though the pressure exerted upon them is equal to that of the surrounding water. By contrast, the gases in the body are compressible, and raising their pressure will decrease their volume. Boyle's law refers to the relationship between volume and pressure, the volume of a gas varying inversely with the pressure exerted upon it. A lung that is half-inflated at a depth of 10 m when the pressure is 2 atm will be fully inflated on the surface. In particular, the air-containing spaces of the head (the nasal and paranasal sinuses, the middle and inner ear spaces) are vulnerable to the effects of Boyle's law as are the spaces within the respiratory system.[1]

The effect of the above is that the reduction in lung volume places a limit on the depth to which an individual can descend in breath-hold diving. The changes in the volume of air in the lungs with alterations in ambient pressure also have implications for divers when assisted by air provided from an external source. In addition there are adverse consequences when sinuses are blocked and pressure cannot be equalized between adjacent internal body cavities. The implications for health and safety are considered in separate sections of this chapter.

Dalton's law concerns the partial pressure of individual gases in a mixture and the partial pressure determines the driving force of a gas moving into the lungs. The partial pressure of each component depends on the proportionate number of molecules present. The sum total of the partial pressures of the individual gases is equal to the total pressure exerted by the gases. Air contains 20.93% O_2, 0.03% CO_2, 79% N_2 while the remainder consists of inert gases, so that the partial pressure of oxygen at a depth of about 40 m (5 atm pressure) is the same as breathing pure oxygen on the surface.

According to Henry's law, the components of a mixture of gases in contact with a liquid will dissolve in direct proportion to their partial pressures. This law is important in both diving and aviation physiology as gases are rapidly absorbed at higher pressures and seek to escape at lower pressures. The resultant adverse effects are known as 'the bends'. These and other consequences of Henry's law are described later.

UNDERWATER STRESS

Water constitutes an alien environment for the recreationist, whether his or her activity is on the surface or underneath it; the risk of drowning is present in either case. As heat is transferred from the body much more rapidly in water than in air, hypothermia is another major hazard in prolonged immersion. The specific heat of water is some thousand-fold greater and its thermal conductivity 25 times greater than air. Consequently, the diver needs thermal protection and so wet suits are used in subaquatic activities in open water to help retain body temperature within the range where thermoregulation is possible. These suits are constructed to have good insulation properties, allowing a thin layer of water to penetrate to the skin which is then warmed whilst the garment protects against further movement of fluid though it.

Prolonged dives demand the supply of oxygen to the individual who has to remain underwater. The depth to which the diver goes determines the external pressure on the body and has numerous physiological repercussions. Lung rupture can occur in indoor swimming pools at a depth of 2 m and people can drown in shallow water. The specific problems are associated with the type of diving and activity involved.

Competitive high diving is a short duration sport where the competitor takes off from a high board to dive into the water. The risks associated with this activity are related to technical faults such as hitting the edge of the board whilst in flight or landing awkwardly in the water. Octopush is a form of hockey played underwater in standard swimming pools. The puck is moved along the pool floor while the players alternate between periods of intense activity underwater and longer recovery bouts swimming on the surface.

The major technological challenges are presented in those activities where hyperbaric factors are involved. These include skin diving and scuba (self contained underwater breathing apparatus) diving, each of which is covered in the sections which follow.

SKIN DIVING

Breath-hold diving was practised 2000 years ago in Greece, Persia, India, Korea and Japan for harvesting pearls and seafood. It was used for warfare purposes in the Mediterranean and Middle Eastern waters even before that time. The technique has also been used for salvaging treasures and is still employed by the Ama women of Korea for a living. More recently, attempts to break new records for depth underwater have led to the growth of competitive breath-hold diving; the common form of recreational activity is known as skin diving.

Skin diving refers to excursions underwater without using artificial aids. The individual's breath-holding ability and pressure changes with increasing depth put a time limit of 2-3 minutes and a depth limit of about 30 m on each dive. The main reasons are the build up of carbon dioxide in the body as metabolism is supported without breathing oxygen whilst, with an increase in depth, the air within the lungs may contract to the point where the O_2 becomes unavailable for gaseous exchange. The usual maximum depth is about 20 m though the international convention is to limit skin diving to 15 m. The Ama, reputed professional pearl divers of Korea and Japan, dive to about 44 m and may perform up to 30 dives in one hour, even in water temperatures as cold as 10°C. In 1969, a US Navy diver performed a breath-hold dive for 148 seconds to a depth of 75 m using only saline-filled goggles and contact lenses as aids in doing so. Seven years later the French diver Jacques Moyel went 102 m below the surface, holding his breath for 219 seconds. In 1999 Umberto

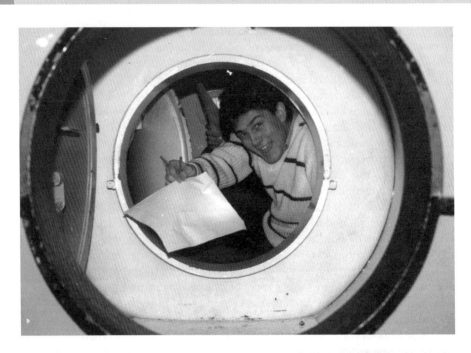

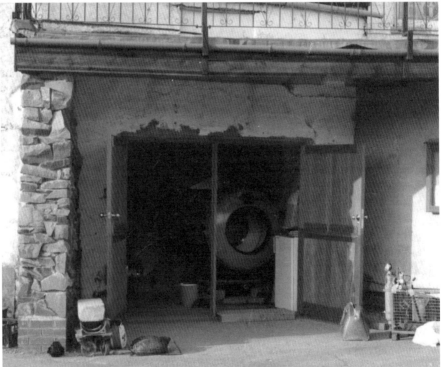

Figure 5.1 Novice diver (above) entering a compression chamber (below) for experience of mood changes at depth

Pellizeri dived to a depth of 150 m. In 2002 Audrey Mestre set a world record of 171 m for free (assisted) diving but died in the attempt to extend it further.[2] She took 102 seconds to reach this depth but drowned as her air bag failed to inflate and bring her to the safety of the surface. Emulation of these exceptional feats should not be attempted by the novice diver for reasons that will shortly become apparent.

The modern history of competitive breath-hold diving began with a recorded dive to 30 m by Raimondo Bucher in 1949. The improvement in this record has been progressive since then even though the duration of the dives remains about 210 seconds. The main reasons for the improvements are the use of counterweights to speed the descent and reduce energy cost, along with assistant devices to accelerate the return to the surface. Inflatable suits, use of hydrodynamic postures and avoidance of redundant movements are part of the strategies used in record attempts. The majority of free divers use fins but no extra weights to dive as deep as possible. Some attempt further depths by employing a metal sled weighing about 90 kg that slides down a steel cable. On deciding it is time to ascend to the surface, the diver releases an air bag that shoots him/her quickly back to the surface. The International Association of Free Divers currently has responsibility for overseeing the sport and certifying records on behalf of its 20,000 participants.

The effort associated with activity underwater leads to a reduction in available oxygen and a build up of carbon dioxide. Changes in the partial pressure of these gases reduce the duration of any breath-hold. In a review of the physiology of extreme breath-hold diving, Ferretti[3] considered that the maximal diving depth is set by the balance between the energy cost of diving, the speed of the dive and the minimal partial pressure of oxygen (PO_2) that is compatible with consciousness on immersion.

Extreme breath-hold divers display a blunted ventilatory response to breathing CO_2 which allows them to attain very low alveolar oxygen (< 30 mmHg) and high alveolar CO_2 (> 50 mmHg) partial pressures at the end of maximal breath-holds in compression chambers (see Figure 5.1). The majority of practitioners of extreme breath-hold diving have experienced loss of consciousness on emersion during their careers, underlining how dangerous the activity is. Awareness of the risks led the World Conference on Underwater Activities to stop recognizing absolute world records and to restrict the rules of assisted breath-hold diving.[3]

The limiting effect of pressure on 'skin diving' can be illustrated by considering its influence on lung volumes. An average diver entering the water would take a maximum inspiration of about 4.5 l. This, together with a residual volume of 1.5 l, would give a total lung volume of 6 l at the surface. Going to a depth of 30 m would cause a fourfold increase in pressure. The air will remain at the same pressure as the surrounding water and tissues and so its volume must be reduced by a decrease in volume of the thoracic cavity (1.5 l in the above example) to equal the residual volume. The residual volume represents the air left in the lungs after a normal exhalation and averages 22-25% of the vital capacity. On the return to the surface the chest re-expands with the reversal of pressure changes.

Any attempt to go lower than a depth that reduces the air in the lungs to a value equal to residual volume is thought to be highly dangerous. If the thoracic volume cannot decrease further, air in the lungs will remain at the same pressure while that of the surrounding tissues and blood will increase with that of the surrounding water. This thoracic squeeze is accompanied by pulmonary oedema, congestion and haemorrhage. Individuals with a very low residual volume and a high total lung capacity can go below the 30 m in this example. It seems also from studies of extreme breath-hold divers that other factors prevent thoracic breakdown at lung volumes less than residual volume. These include alterations in heart, lungs and the dome of the diaphragm muscle that are associated with the redistribution of blood from the body's periphery.[3]

Similarly, if the links between the sinuses and the respiratory system or the Eustachian tubes are obstructed, it is impossible to equalize pressure during the dive by moving air into the middle ear and so excessive pain and physical injury such as rupture of the ear drum may occur. Consequently, an ability to clear the ears to equalize pressure in the middle ear with that of the external ear is essential. This is relatively easy to achieve in practice by such manoeuvres as swallowing, pinching one's nose or breathing forcefully against a closed epiglottis. It is essential to be free from acute or chronic infections of the respiratory tract. Nor should divers use ear plugs as these may simply be forced into the aural canals. If goggles or helmets are worn, these must have facilities for equalizing the pressure within to that of the water outside.

The other limit to breath-holding time is linked with the change in partial pressure of respiratory gases, specifically the increased PCO_2 in alveolar gas and arterial blood and the fall in PO_2. It is possible to extend breath-holding time by hyperventilating beforehand; this manoeuvre washes out the CO_2 from the alveoli and delays the eventual stimulation of the respiratory centre by its reaccumulation. The diver may lose consciousness because of a lack of oxygen before the rising CO_2 is high enough to force the diver to the surface for a breath of air. Alternatively, when the increase in PCO_2 promotes the urge to rebreathe and the diver begins to ascend towards the water surface, the falling pressure of the gases that is associated with ascent may cause a drop in PO_2 to the point where consciousness may be lost. Death by drowning then quickly follows. For these reasons the practice among spear fishermen and skin divers of hyperventilating prior to going underwater is to be condemned.

Skin diving equipment is mostly restricted to simple masks and fins, while a snorkel tube may be used for breathing near the surface. Tortoise shell, suitably ground and polished, formed a primitive mask which was used historically by pearl divers in the Persian Gulf and in Polynesian waters. There are in excess of 150 types of mask commercially available to today's divers, though most are sold to scuba divers. Specifications for masks and snorkels are contained in the British Standards Institute's lists of standards and amendment slips.

For many centuries, primitive tubes for breathing underwater were familiar to Indians in Central America and to Greenland's Eskimos, and were the precursors of the varieties of snorkel used today. The limits to snorkelling are set firstly by the fact that the snorkel adds to the dead space in ventilation and when this pulmonary dead space is about 60% of the total lung volume, adequate gas exchange becomes impossible. Secondly, the compressive force of water against the chest cavity means that at a depth of only 1 m the inspiratory muscles are unable to overcome external pressure and expand thoracic dimensions so that inspiration is impossible without air supplied at an increased pressure. These considerations mean that the snorkel size is normally limited to about 46 cm in length with a bore of 22 mm, although the maximum length of the tube measured along its central line from the flange of the mouthpiece to the upper opening is 60 cm in the British Standards specification and the internal diameter is between 15 and 22.5 mm.

The difficulties associated with vision underwater and selection of appropriate ameliorative masks, goggles and lenses are covered in various specialist texts (for example Miles and MacKay,[4] Bennett and Elliott[5]). Masks that incorporate safety glass are recommended to avoid their destruction on hard underwater objects. Other risks to the skin diver include getting cut on sharp coral edges, mishandling of harpoons, spear guns or a hand spear, and incurring injury of varying severity from marine life.

SCUBA DIVING

The restrictions of breath-holding and increasing pressure at depth are overcome with apparatus that ensures a continuous supply of air, or other breathing mixture, at a pressure equal to that of the water in which the diver is operating. In standard conventional or 'hard-hat' diving, the individual wore an armoured helmet, breast-plate and weighted suit and was supplied with air from a hose fed by means of a compressor on the surface. The 'ventilated helmet' has been in regular use for over a century and is still one of the safest and simplest types of apparatus available. One of the problems associated with its use is the lack of mobility due to the hose from the surface. Self-contained underwater breathing apparatus permits the diver a free flow of air for a sustained period with equipment that is not excessively heavy underwater, permitting good mobility. The apparatus may be in the form of an open circuit system (expired gases are discharged into the water) or a closed circuit (expired gases are not discharged). In the closed system, expired CO_2 is absorbed in soda lime canisters and the oxygen is re-circulated. This system is unsuitable at depths below 8-10 m because of a risk of oxygen toxicity. It is also imperative that the CO_2 is completely absorbed to prevent its recirculation, which could cause CO_2 poisoning. It is suitable for diving in confined spaces such as underground caves. The self-contained open circuit system is widely used for recreation purposes, gases being supplied by means of a demand valve from compressed air cylinders carried on the diver's back: in this case, the exhaled gases are vented into the water, leaving a characteristic trail of bubbles. The regulator valve through which the air flows reduces the pressure of the gas to that of the particular depth of the diver. A slight negative pressure is created as the diver inspires, causing the demand valve to open and release air to the diver. This valve closes on exhalation as the air is discharged into the water.

The nitrogen and oxygen supplied in air are both soluble in the blood of the diver and diffuse throughout the body's tissues. As is the case when breathing on dry land at sea-level, the oxygen and nitrogen dissolved in the tissues are in equilibrium with the partial pressure of those gases in the lungs. As air is supplied at increased pressure at depth, the greater partial pressures of the two gases in the lung drive more of each into the blood and tissues. Any effects of these gases on physiological and psychological functions as well as the effects of the alterations in pressure and volume must be considered if the safety of the diver is to be secured. These changes and the appropriate counter-measures are now summarized.

CONSEQUENCES OF WORKING UNDER WATER

Pressure and volume changes

The relationship between pressure and volume described by Boyle's law operates in the same way for the scuba diver as for the skin diver. The pressure of the surrounding water controls the pressure at which the demand valves supply air to the diver from the cylinders carried on his back. At depth, the pressure of gas delivered (at the higher ambient pressure) is greater than that released at the surface, so that the deeper a diver operates, the shorter is the life of the supply cylinder. The rate of use and available supply must be carefully monitored by the diver and the capacity of the cylinders dictates the duration of the dive.

A great deal more air can be carried in liquid form than as compressed gas, and this has led to the development of cryogenic gear for deep sea professionals. This system uses liquid air at extremely low temperatures, is relatively light and can extend the time that a given cylinder lasts. The very low liquid air temperature is raised by a heat exchanger while a pressure regulator alters the pressure according to the temperature and pressure of the surrounding water. Though this system has potential for the sports diver, the high cost limits its use.

Density

As changes in the pressure of gas cause proportionate changes in its density, air breathed at a depth of 10 m is twice as dense and viscous as that breathed on the surface. This calls for increased effort by the respiratory muscles to move this air into and out of the lungs because of the increased resistance of the denser air in the respiratory tract. A conscious effort may be needed to overcome this extra resistance in order to avoid retention of CO_2 and get enough O_2. The experienced diver tends to control his or her breathing pattern and to avoid short bursts of intense physical activity of the type performed by sports participants on dry land or by 'octopush' (a sport resembling hockey under water) players in shallow water. The problems presented by changes in density are overcome for the professional diver who has to operate at great depth by having the nitrogen in the air breathed replaced with a much lighter gas. Helium is usually the gas used for this purpose unless great depths are being explored.

Nitrogen narcosis

The use of helium confers a further advantage. More nitrogen is dissolved in the blood and diffuses into the tissues with increasing depth because of its greater partial pressure in inhaled air. Nitrogen has a pronounced narcotic effect on the central nervous system which is sometimes referred to as 'raptures of the deep'. The result is a deterioration in function with a slowing of mental processes and intellectual function.[6,7] These changes can be induced in a compression chamber at an equivalent ambient pressure of 40 m depth (see Figure 5.1).

Sensations of euphoria are first felt at about 30 m, although there is considerable variation between individuals. The safety limit for a scuba diver who is largely responsible for his own security is about 50 m because of narcosis. The commercial 'Standard Diver' with helmet and heavy boots may go much deeper, as his safety is totally dependent upon the surface attendants who pump air down and can pull the diver up in an emergency. Nevertheless, the diver's skills are adversely affected with increasing depth.

Helium is less narcotic than nitrogen and so is used by deep diving professionals in an oxyhelium mixture at depths beyond 50 m. The effects of breathing oxygen-helium mixtures on physiological functions were extensively explored some decades ago (e.g. Baddeley and Fleming,[8] Bennett and Towse[9]). Oxyhelium tends to be used by professionals down to a depth of about 300 m. One side-effect of helium is a gross distortion in speech, making verbal communication in high pressure chambers difficult. It also increases heat loss from the body. Helium begins to induce narcotic symptoms beyond a depth of about 420 m. Memory impairment has also been reported during a deep dive aided by helium,[6] providing concern about the appropriate oxyhelium mixture to be used at great depth.

Oxygen toxicity

Oxygen is poisonous if breathed in its pure form for several hours on the surface. Underwater, more of it is dissolved in blood and tissues so that the threshold of oxygen toxicity occurs earlier. For example, a 20 min exposure to

Table 5.1 Effects of oxygen poisoning on the central nervous system in normal men[5]

Physiological effects	Behaviour	Subjective effects
Bradycardia	Clumsiness	Apprehension
Palpitations	Convulsions	Choking sensation
Respiratory changes:	Fidgeting	Depression
hiccoughs, panting	Lip twitching	Euphoria
Spasmodic vomiting	Syncope	Nausea
Sweating		Sleepiness
Visual symptoms:		Unpleasant sensations:
loss of acuity		gustatory
constricted visual field		olfactory

pure oxygen at 10 m depth produces lip twitching and convulsions (see Table 5.1). Consequently, use of pure oxygen is limited to very shallow depths; it is unacceptable for sports divers, though it may be used by cavers to pass through flooded links between caves. Use of nitrox (a mixture of O_2 and N_2) or oxygen-enriched air poses a similar threat of oxygen toxicity at depths of even less than 50 m.

As the partial pressure of oxygen increases with depth, the PO_2 of a normal air mixture eventually becomes toxic. At about 100 m oxygen poisoning becomes a real risk because the partial pressure of oxygen is now 11 times that at the surface. The risk is avoided by lowering the percentage of oxygen in the breathing mixture to achieve an acceptable PO_2. This means that at a depth of 200 m, a concentration of 4% oxygen in helium is acceptable.[1]

Carbon dioxide poisoning

Carbon dioxide toxicity is usually associated with the use of closed-circuit systems beyond the point when the absorbent (usually soda lime) is totally saturated. Some experienced divers using open-circuit breathing apparatus are known to become 'CO_2 retainers'.[10] The increased CO_2 threshold may be a helpful adaptation but can act synergistically with other factors to cause unconsciousness underwater.

High pressure neurological syndrome

In the mid-1960s it was noted that during so-called bounce dives to 243 m at a compression rate of 30 m/min, divers experienced coarse tremors, nausea and vomiting. The gross tremors have a major component between 8 Hz and 12 Hz and may be noticed at depths as shallow as 140 m depending on the ambient temperature and the compression rate. Cerebral effects include microsleeps, decreases in the percentage of alpha waves and an increase in the percentage of theta waves in the EEG. The syndrome causes severe incapacitation between 420 and 550 m depth, even at very slow compression rates which virtually eliminate the direct effects of compression, and so seems to be related to the hydrostatic pressure. It was referred to as 'high pressure neurological syndrome' (HPNS) by Brauer and colleagues.[11] Hydrostatic pressure acts upon all membranes in a manner that allows the convulsions of HPNS to be partially compensated for by the absorption of an inert gas.

The syndrome has been subjected to extensive investigation, leading to greater and greater depths and pressures being explored in open water and in simulations. A detailed account of the early investigations was presented by Bennett.[12] One study at Duke University involved a 28-day stay in a compression chamber; for 4 days the simulated depth was 650 m and for 24 hours it was 686 m. It was possible to carry out extensive physiological investigations involving venepuncture at 650 m, whilst one of the subjects was able to cycle for 5 minutes on an ergometer at 240 W.

The studies at Duke University and elsewhere have shown that the effects of HPNS can be ameliorated by slow and staged compression rates to permit adaptation. The value of using trimix – a mixture of helium, nitrogen and oxygen – rather than oxyhelium in suppressing HPNS has also been demonstrated. Brauer et al.[11] have shown that nitrous oxide or hydrogen was also effective in preventing HPNS in mice. Research to ascertain the optimal compression schedules and the best and safest gas mixtures continues; Bennett[12] concluded that, '…as in the past, the desire of some to impose depth limitations on diving may continue to be confounded by the solutions provided by careful and ingenious research'.

DECOMPRESSION

Problems associated with decompression may arise in the course of returning to the surface. During descent, the gases breathed pass through the blood and tissues until ultimately a new equilibrium is established, after which no further net transfer occurs. The absorbing gases can only enter the body through the lungs during this period but when the pressure is released during the final ascent the resulting decrease in pressure applies throughout the body. The dissolved gases – oxygen, nitrogen and helium in the case of deep divers – must come out of solution. The rate of delivery of blood to the lungs and the amount released by the blood as it passes through the pulmonary capillary bed may be insufficient to stop the excess gas coming out of solution in different parts of the body and forming bubbles. As the consequences can be dire, it is essential that the ascent is controlled to allow excess gases time to leave via the lungs (see Figure 5.2).

It is possible for the sport diver, operating within the range of depths used

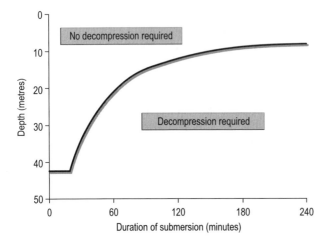

Figure 5.2 Time schedules for decompression depend on both the depth and duration of the dive[2]

for recreation, to surface directly provided that the time spent at the bottom is short. Divers stick to established codes of practice and generally abide by the compression tables available to all sub-aqua clubs. Time limits for decompression are illustrated in Figure 5.2. The tables lay down the number of stops, their duration and the stage of ascent of the diver. They accommodate calculations for decompression schedules in cases of repeated dives.

A great deal of time must be spent in decompression in cases of deep and lengthy dives. Among commercial divers the fact that a new equilibrium of saturation with gas under pressure is eventually attained is exploited; the diver may then remain at that depth for many weeks. This allows professionals to operate from pressurized cabins for sustained spells, at the end of which a single, albeit prolonged, decompression routine suffices. It has been suggested that this form of so-called 'saturation diving' may have application if pressurized underwater holiday camps in undersea areas like the Australian Barrier Reef become a tourist attraction.[1]

There is a wide range of injuries and illnesses associated with faulty decompression. The first risk is pulmonary barotrauma, or burst lung, which can occur when ascent is too rapid. The air confined in the chest at depth is compressed. As the surface is approached its pressure falls and volume increases (Boyle's law). As the diver relaxes the chest muscles, the sudden expansion and escape of air may tear lung tissue. This allows air to pass into the surrounding tissue, producing emphysema or air emboli which enter the circulation and may block vital arteries to the heart or brain. The treatment is instant repressurisation in a decompression chamber or return to depth in water if this facility is unavailable.[1]

Formation of air bubbles on ascent can lead to various symptoms; the most common is pain in the joints and limbs which is usually referred to as 'the bends'. The 'bends' describes severe pain, minor pain around the joints being known as 'niggles'. 'Staggers' refers to involvement of the spinal cord or brain with varying levels of muscular or sensory paralysis. Permanent disability may result from bubbles being released within the brain or spinal cord and careful therapeutic decompression is called for. 'Chokes' refers to respiratory distress associated with bubble formation within the pulmonary alveolar circulation, though in this case recompression is not essential. Finally, bone necrosis at the end of long bones, which may cause severe arthritis, can occur some time after exposure, though this happens to the professional rather than the recreational diver.

Surface decompression procedures have been employed as a cost-cutting exercise among professional divers. The diver is brought to the surface and almost immediately transferred to a decompression chamber. Although there are few immediate observable symptoms when using this procedure, long-term problems associated with miniature bubble formation are likely. In particular, damage to nerve and bone cells can occur when bubbles are formed within these tissues. Such adverse effects may remain latent for months or even years, but are immediately evident with contemporary medical and imaging techniques.

CAVE DIVING

Diving in caves can be a recreational activity or a professional requirement, for example for public health rescue teams or underground cave cartographers. An underground cave network may be comprised of a large number of interconnecting passages, in the main partly but some totally underwater, possessing their own myriad of gloomy recesses. Apart from the potential risk of hypothermia and physiological problems linked with compression, there are specific considerations in this activity.

The duration of the dives needs to be planned so that the team takes an adequate supply of air on the underground trip. The divers must lay down a nylon guidance line as they enter the cave, with indicators of the direction of travel: this procedure is necessary in case of getting disorientated and losing sense of direction. Caves may be dark and murky and so the use of lamps is mandatory. Cave divers employ special 'kicks' as they swim to avoid disturbing silt beneath them. Exhaled bubbles may also interfere with visibility.

Swimming through underground caves is costly in terms of energy and the oxygen supply carried by the cave diver is limited. These divers may use battery-powered underwater scooters which can pull them quickly through the water, thereby saving their energy and stretching their air supply. The divers must always allow a margin for safety in case of contingencies and be continually vigilant about time elapsed. In common with sports divers, the 'caver' at depth will have impaired proprioception due to the increased buoyancy in water and so become subject to disorientation during unforeseen episodes. Whilst the coastal diver may have to pay attention to dangerous marine life, the cave diver needs to be careful of jutting edges on cave walls or protruding stalagmites and stalactites.

HYPERBARIC EXERCISE

There has been some research interest in determining exercise capabilities in water. Mobile underwater ergometers permit control and measurement of divers' work output during swimming at ocean depths up to 30 m and have become highly reliable during extended use.[13] A more specific test than cycle ergometry uses a drag board which introduces a reproducible resistance to the swimming diver.[14] A standard exercise can be presented by controlling the resistance and the swimming speed.

Obtaining physiological measurements in sub-aquatic activities is technically demanding. A system for accurate measurement of oxygen intake ($\dot{V}O_2$) at different depths and exercise intensities was described by Dwyer.[13] He also developed a system for simultaneous measurement of ventilation, respiratory rate, tidal volume and the ECG during dives in open water.

Measurement of physiological variables in compression chambers is also very difficult. It requires extensive specialist facilities and skilled personnel. Nevertheless, Bennett[12] demonstrated that exercise studies could be conducted in simulated dives of 650 m depth, during which respiratory and arterial blood analyses were performed.

The metabolic load on the underwater diver may be affected by the temperature as well as the pressure of the surrounding water. There is also an increased heat loss when helium is breathed. As the temperature of the water becomes cooler with depth and the wet suit material worn by the diver is also increasingly compressed, so losing its insulation properties, maintenance of body temperature may require an increased oxygen intake. The increased compression of the wet suit may also adversely affect the mobility of the diver. Another factor is that the diver's equipment can increase the drag and so affect the individual's muscular efficiency in moving through the water. Swim fins have been designed to assist the motion of the body through the water but require metabolic energy to use. Ease of performance underwater can be assisted by reducing the energy requirement associated with fin use. McMurray[15] showed that vented super-fins which direct water flow were superior to conventional fins for underwater work. He also noted that the surface area and flexibility of the swim fins were important features in their design.

The diver's performance underwater is, therefore, influenced by a number of factors dictated by the environment to which he or she is exposed and the equipment used. The individual's exercise capacity is affected by the muscular efficiency, thermoregulatory state and metabolic loading. The most important physiological factors are probably the ability to tolerate high levels of CO_2 and the percentage of the $\dot{V}O_{2\ max}$ (or relative exercise intensity) that can be sustained before a critical PCO_2 is reached.

FITNESS FOR DIVING

According to Elliott,[10] professional divers – particularly the sports diving instructor upon whom the life of a trainee in an underwater emergency may depend – should be expected to have the highest standard of physical, medical and mental fitness. The criteria should be strict, since cardiopulmonary and other important functional requirements are subject to deterioration with age. Less strict criteria may be applied to amateur divers who are free to choose when or where to engage in diving activities.

Furthermore, there are contraindications to diving that would render the activity temporarily unsuitable. These include any upper respiratory tract infections, any Eustachian tube obstructions that would impair the equalization of pressure in the middle ear, any impediments to mobility or dexterity, and any peripheral circulatory disease that limits exercise tolerance. A comprehensive list of contraindications to sports scuba diving was published by Elliott.[10] Diving is not advised during pregnancy or intended pregnancy.

OVERVIEW

The human's ability to develop technologies to cope with adverse environmental conditions is reflected in human records for diving achievements in deep water. Detailed description of the risks involved, possible only after the most careful scrutiny, has laid the foundation for setting out guidelines for safety and training practices. Simulators may be used to enhance training practices though development of appropriate equipment becomes increasingly important as stresses become extreme. It is also important to consider possible interactions with other environmental stressors such as cold and hypoxia. The adaptations to hypoxia may have residual effects for the diver which would exacerbate the risks associated with hyperbaric pressure. Consequently, diving manuals quite rightly advise against diving after recreational activity such as skiing at altitude or after airflight which involves descent from a low pressure environment. It is also important to avoid strenuous exercise or air flight immediately after diving in case of air bubble formation due to the lowered ambient pressure.

References

1. Reilly T, Miles S. Background to injuries in swimming and diving. In: Sports fitness and sports injuries. Reilly T (ed). London: Faber and Faber, 1981:159-167
2. McCrory P. The big blue. Brit J Sports Med 2003; 37,1
3. Ferretti G. Extreme human breath-hold diving. Europ J Appl Physiol 2001; 84:254-271
4. Miles S, Mackay DE. Underwater medicine. London: Adiard Coles, 1976
5. Bennett P, Elliott DH. The physiology and medicine of diving. London: Balliere Tindall, 1982
6. Biersner RJ, Cameron BJ. Memory impairment during a deep helium dive. Aerospace Med 1970; 41:658-661
7. Thomas V, Reilly T. Effects of compression on human performance and affective states. Brit J Sports Med 1974; 8:188-190

8. Baddeley AD, Flemming NC. The efficiency of divers breathing oxygen-helium. Ergonomics 1967; 10:311-319

9. Bennett P, Towse EJ. Performance efficiency of man breathing oxygen-helium at depths between 100 feet and 1500 feet. Aerospace Med 1971; 42:1147-1156

10. Elliott D. The underwater environment. In: Oxford textbook of sports medicine. Harries M, Williams C, Stanish W et al. (eds). Oxford: Oxford Medical Publications, 1998:225-229

11. Brauer RW, Goldman SM, Beaver RW et al. N_2, H_2 and N_2O antagonism of high pressure neurological syndrome in mice. Undersea Biomed Res 1974; 1:59-72

12. Bennett P. The high pressure nervous syndrome in man. In: The physiology and medicine of diving. Bennett P, Elliott DH (eds). London: Balliere Tindall, 1982:262-296

13. Dwyer J. Measurement of oxygen consumption in scuba divers working in open water. Ergonomics 1977; 20:377-388

14. Pilmanis AA, Henriksen J, Dwyer HJ. An underwater ergometer for diver work performance in the ocean. Ergonomics 1977; 20:51-55

15. McMurray RG. Comparative effects of conventional and super-swimfin design. Hum Factors 1977; 19:495-501

Chapter 6

The stress of travel

CHAPTER CONTENTS

Introduction 89
Daily rhythms and the role of the body clock 90
Travel fatigue – the effects of long-distance flights with little change in the time zone 95

Rapid transitions across time zones – jet lag 96
Advice regarding jet lag 103
Slow transitions across time zones 111
Overview 113

INTRODUCTION

Competitive sport is now recognized on a global scale and people at many levels, from the Olympic athlete to the recreational runner, have the opportunity of competing abroad. Travelling to strange places for purposes of competing in sport might seem attractive; in reality it is stressful and makes great demands on all concerned, demands that might include mental as well as physiological disturbances.

Any long journey, nowadays generally by plane, will result in the traveller suffering from a group of symptoms during the day of travel, and perhaps the day after, which may be called 'travel fatigue'. For those on journeys that take an extended period of time (yachtsmen sailing the Atlantic, for example) the problem is also one of sleep loss, and this will be covered at the end of the chapter. If a journey entails crossing several time zones rapidly, then there is a longer-lasting group of symptoms popularly known as 'jet lag', sleep loss being one of its components. While suffering from jet lag, individuals perform sub-optimally, partly due to this sleep loss.

The complex problems involved in these stressful circumstances become simpler to study if the components due to travel fatigue, jet lag and sleep loss are separated. The comparatively new science of chronobiology provides us with an understanding of many of these different components.

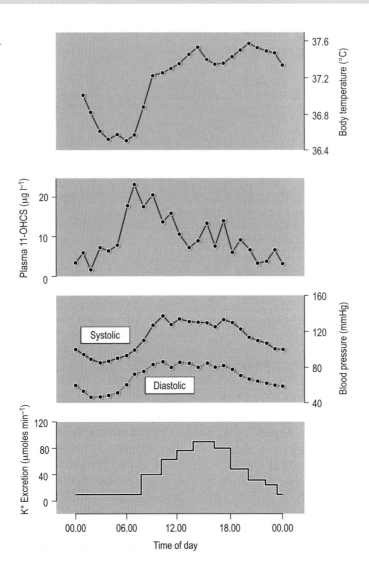

Figure 6.1 Some circadian rhythms in a subject sleeping from 24:00 to 08:00 h[2]

DAILY RHYTHMS AND THE ROLE OF THE BODY CLOCK

Chronobiology is the study of how living organisms respond to environmental time, whether this is a solar day (24 h), a lunar day (24.8 h), the monthly changes in the height of tides, or seasonal (yearly) changes. Daily rhythms are the most widespread and obvious, and the field is surveyed in Reilly et al.[1]

In subjects living normally (asleep at night and active in the daytime), core temperature shows higher values in the daytime and lower values at night. Peak temperatures are observed around 16:00-20:00 h, and lowest values

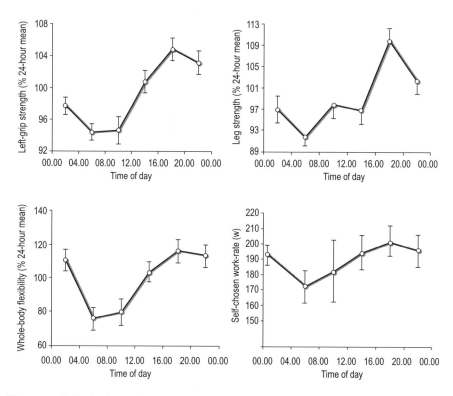

Figure 6.2 Daily rhythms of grip strength,[1] isometric knee extension,[1] whole-body flexibility,[1] and self-selected work-rate[3]

about 04:00-06:00 h. Many other variables, including heart rate, mental performance, self-chosen work-rate, and several components of physical performance, show rhythms that are timed similarly. By contrast, for many hormones and for the perceived exertion associated with mental or physical tasks, the observed rhythm is the inverse, with nocturnal values being higher than those in the daytime (Figures 6.1 and 6.2).

These results might indicate that the body is merely responding to a day-orientated society, with opportunity at night for sleep and recuperation. Such an explanation is only partially correct, however, as can be deduced from studies of an individual during a 'constant routine'. In this protocol, the subjects are required to stay awake and sedentary for at least 24 hours in an environment of constant temperature, humidity and lighting. They also need to engage in similar activities throughout, generally reading or listening to music, and to take identical meals at regularly-spaced intervals. In spite of the fact that this protocol means that any rhythmicity due to the environment and lifestyle has been removed, the rhythm of core temperature (and other variables that have been studied) persists, even though its amplitude is decreased (Figure 3).

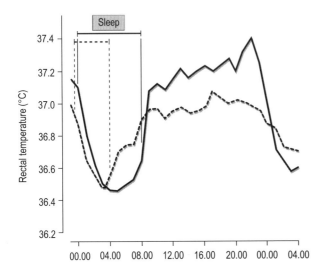

Figure 6.3 Mean circadian changes in core (rectal) temperature measured hourly in 8 subjects: living normally and sleeping from 24:00 to 08:00 h (solid line); and then woken at 04:00 h and spending the next 24 h on a 'constant routine' (dashed line)[4]

The rhythm that remains must arise within the body; its generation is attributed to the 'body clock'. Effects of the environment and lifestyle are present, however, as can be deduced from the finding that the amplitude of the rhythm has decreased. This component of the rhythm is termed 'exogenous', to distinguish it from the 'endogenous' component due to the body clock. In subjects living a conventional lifestyle, these two components are in phase (Figure 6.3). Thus, during the daytime, body temperature is raised by the body clock acting in synchrony with the alerting effects of the environment and physical and mental activities; during the night, the clock, environment and inactivity all act to lower body temperature.

The site of the body clock and its circadian nature

Humans have paired groups of cells in the base of the hypothalamus, a region of the brain closely associated with temperature regulation, the release of hormones, appetite for food and sleep. These cells are called the suprachiasmatic nuclei (SCN).[5] One piece of evidence (there are many others) that this is the site of the clock is that cells from the SCN show a daily rhythmicity in nerve activity when they are cultured *in vitro* in constant conditions; no other cells from the brain show autonomous activity in such circumstances.

When humans are studied in an environment in which there are no time cues – in an underground cave, for example – the daily rhythms of sleep and waking, body temperature, hormone release, and so on, continue. This fact confirms their endogenous origin, but it is observed that the period of such rhythms is closer to 25 than 24 hours. As a result of this, the subject becomes progressively more delayed with respect to the outside environment. For this reason, these clock-driven rhythms are called circadian (from the Latin for 'about a day').

Recent work upon many species of plants and animals, including humans, has shown that there is a large degree of evolutionary conservation with regard to clock mechanisms, their molecular biochemistry and genetics. Briefly (see Clayton et al.[6]), a group of 'clock genes' is transcribed to form mRNA which is then translated by the cytoplasmic ribosomes to make 'clock proteins'. These proteins are responsible for many of the rhythmic processes (neural activity, transmitter production, and so on) associated with the clock functions of the SCN cells. After modification in the cytoplasm, some of these proteins move back into the nucleus where they inhibit the transcription of the clock genes. As a result, the production of clock proteins begins to decline. In turn, this results in a loss of inhibition of DNA transcription, and so the clock genes are transcribed once more. The whole cycle takes about 24 hours to accomplish, thereby accounting for the circadian nature of the body clock.

Adjustment of the body clock

Such circadian rhythmicity implies that the body clock needs to be adjusted continually for it to remain synchronized to a solar (24-h) day and if it is to provide useful information about the passage of time. Synchrony is achieved by 'zeitgebers' (German for 'time-givers'): rhythms resulting, directly or indirectly, from the environment. In different mammals, rhythms of the light-dark cycle, of food availability-unavailability, of activity-inactivity, and of social influences, act singly or in combination. In humans, a combination of these zeitgebers is normally present, although the most important are the regular nocturnal release of melatonin and the light-dark cycle.

Melatonin is the hormone secreted by the pineal gland,[7] and its secretion is closely linked with the rhythm of core temperature. In the evening, its secretion increases at the same time as the core temperature is falling, and, in the morning, the end of secretion of this hormone and the rise of core temperature occur simultaneously. Melatonin has several effects upon the body, amongst which is a vasodilatation that increases heat loss.[8] In the evening, therefore, core temperature falls due to the direct effects of melatonin secretion being superimposed upon the heat loss that results from the body clock resetting the 'set-point' of thermoregulation to a lower value. In the morning, the rise in set-point (due to the body clock) and the termination of melatonin secretion both act to raise core temperature.

Light acts as a zeitgeber because its effect upon the body clock depends on the time at which the individual is exposed to it.[9,10] Pulses of bright light (that is, light of an intensity found outdoors rather than domestically) that are centred in the 6-hour 'window' immediately after the trough of the body temperature rhythm (the trough normally being 03:00-05:00 h, see Figures 6.1 and 6.3) produce a phase advance; pulses centred in the 6-h window before the temperature minimum, a phase delay; those centred away from the trough by more than a few hours have little effect. Light pulses that are weaker (and similar in intensity to domestic lighting) also affect the clock but produce smaller phase shifts.[11,12] This observation is important, since most humans have very little exposure to natural daylight.

In practice, therefore, exposure to light on waking in the morning, and even to light passing through our eyelids when asleep at this time, will cause a small advance of the body clock. This response will result in the circadian clock becoming synchronized to the solar day.

Ingestion of melatonin can also advance or delay the body clock, according to the time at which it is ingested.[13] The shifts produced at a particular time are in the opposite direction to those produced by light exposure at that time. Thus, melatonin in the afternoon and evening tends to advance the body clock and, in the morning, to delay it. Melatonin is sometimes called an 'internal zeitgeber'. Receptors for melatonin have been found in the SCN, and are believed to be the means by which it acts upon the body clock.

Since bright light inhibits melatonin secretion, the phase-shifting effects of light and melatonin reinforce each other. Bright light in the early morning, just after the temperature minimum, advances the phase of the body clock – not only directly but also indirectly, since it suppresses melatonin secretion and so prevents the phase-delaying effect that melatonin would have exerted at this time.[14]

When light acts as a zeitgeber, information passes to the SCN from the eyes via a direct pathway, the retinohypothalamic tract. It seems that the retinae contain a sub-group of receptors whose visual pigment is based on vitamin B_2 (rather than the more conventional vitamin A-based opsins), and it is this sub-group that is responsible for the light signals going to the SCN.[15] The light signal appears to act via an excitatory amino acid such as glutamate and induction of immediate early genes.

An additional input pathway to the SCN via the intergeniculate leaflet exists, this probably being for non-photic zeitgebers (activity, for example) as evidenced in studies of hamsters. In humans also, this pathway is present and might act as a means for enabling a general rhythmic flux of 'excitement', whether derived from mental, physical or social rhythms, to act as a zeitgeber.

The role of the body clock

The body clock produces rhythmicity in the hypothalamus and nearby regions of the brain. Since these areas control temperature regulation, hormone release, feeding and sleep, it can be seen that the body as a whole will become rhythmic. The effects of the clock are two-fold. First, they enable physical and mental activity and their associated biochemical and cardiovascular changes to be promoted in the daytime, and actions involving recovery and restitution during a period of inactivity to be promoted at night. The second role of the body clock is to enable preparations to be made for the switches from the active to the sleeping state, and vice versa. Such changes require that a whole series of biochemical and physiological functions be set in motion before the actual events of falling asleep or waking up take place.

This rhythmicity due to the body clock is of direct relevance to travellers and to athletes.[1] The abilities to fall asleep and to stay asleep are controlled by the body clock, being easier when core temperature is falling (in the evening) or low (in the night). When awake, individuals' adrenaline secretion, muscle strength, short-term maximal power output and self-chosen work rate are all greatest at about 18:00 h (when core temperature is around its peak). At about this time also, many aspects of mental and physical performance are at their best (Figure 6.2), and the perceived exertion for a given amount of physical and mental activity is felt to be least. Most personal best performances in sport are set at this time.

This knowledge will help an understanding of some of the problems associated with travel. First, the effects of a flight over a long distance but not crossing time zones, from the UK to South Africa, for example, will be considered. Such flights cause travel fatigue but not what has come to be termed 'jet lag'.

TRAVEL FATIGUE – THE EFFECTS OF LONG–DISTANCE FLIGHTS WITH LITTLE CHANGE IN THE TIME ZONE

Travel fatigue is caused in part by the worry associated with preparations for the flights, the flights themselves, and becoming attuned to the new environment. Major contributory factors during flights include boredom, a prolonged period spent in a cramped posture, sleep loss and the dry cabin air. The symptoms are essentially over within 48 hours, provided appropriate remedial action is taken.[1]

Before the flight

Preparations for the journey include ensuring that the passport is valid and that any visa requirements have been met, that health advice (including any inoculations that might be required) has been sought and acted upon, that the individual has sufficient funds and clothing for the trip, and that appropriate medication that might be required has been packed. Many of these preparations can be done well in advance so that problems do not arise if delays occur or if more time is required for extra security arrangements. Preparations also include arranging the flight or flights, and often choices can be made about whether to fly by day or by night. For professional athletes and sports teams, these arrangements tend to be made by the group's management personnel which removes some of the hassles of planning the trip for the individuals concerned.

During the flight

During the flight, several problems arise. The flight cabin is a cramped area, and it provides only a very limited opportunity for movement. Being immobile for extended periods of time increases the risk of developing cramp and even, with air travel of more than four hours, deep-vein thrombosis in susceptible individuals. Passengers are advised to walk around the cabin and to do some stretching exercises if there is opportunity. In addition, isometric exercises in the seat can liven up a sluggish circulation, and the wearing of support stockings might be beneficial.

A further problem arises because the cabin air is very dry; this low humidity can cause lips to become sore and also lead to a dry mouth and throat, and to a general dehydration. Sore lips can be avoided by the use of lip salve, and dehydration by increasing fluid intake. However, alcoholic drinks, tea or coffee are not ideal since they tend to cause further dehydration due to their diuretic effects; spring water, soft drinks and fruit juice are all more suitable. Making a suitable drink part of the cabin luggage is a good precautionary measure. It has also been suggested that the recirculation of cabin air during a flight could contribute to an increased incidence of upper respiratory tract infection.

For those who wear contact lenses, the eyes can become sore. In these circumstances, wearing spectacles instead is recommended.

There is always the problem of deciding how to pass the time on a long flight. Sleeping or napping is advised only at times that correspond to night-time at the destination. (Where long-haul flights incorporate two or three legs with brief stop-overs in transit and a total journey around 24 hours, a sleep *en route* at night-time in the immediate environment of the plane would be acceptable.) If too much sleep is taken during the daytime, the traveller might find it difficult to sleep at night after arrival at the destination.

After the flight

After arrival, baggage has to be collected, customs must be cleared, and the final destination must be reached, all of which take time and can cause aggravation, particularly if there are problems. When the destination is reached, the natural tendency is to sleep because of fatigue. This is a good idea only if it is night-time; normally, it is daytime, and so a recuperative nap of no more than about 1 hour, followed by an invigorating shower and a relaxing drink, is recommended.

By the next day, the effects of travel fatigue will have worn off. The traveller can work or train well, or enjoy the holiday.

The problems and advice to travellers are summarized in Box 6.1.

RAPID TRANSITIONS ACROSS TIME ZONES – JET LAG

To achieve the above aims, the body clock needs to be stable and robust, and not to respond to transient changes in the environment or lifestyle of the individual. For example, a clock that rapidly adjusted would compromise the phasing of the circadian rhythms of an animal during an eclipse of the sun, of an individual who woke transiently in the night, or of a person who took a nap in the daytime. The observation that the body clock is, in fact, slow to

Box 6.1 Checklist for travel fatigue[16]

Symptoms:
Fatigue
Disorientation
Headaches
'Travel weariness'

Causes:
Disruption of normal routine
Hassles associated with travel (checking in/baggage claim/customs clearance)
Dehydration due to dry cabin air

Advice:
Before the journey:
Plan the journey well in advance
Try to arrange for any stop-over to be comfortable
Make sure about documentation, inoculations, visas
Make arrangements at your destination

On the plane:
Take some roughage (e.g. apples) to eat
Drink plenty of water or fruit juice (rather than tea/coffee/alcohol)

On reaching the destination:
Relax with a non-alcoholic drink
Take a shower
Take a *brief* nap, if required.

adjust to changes in lifestyle makes sound ecological sense, therefore.

However, such an intransigence becomes the bane of those who undergo time-zone transitions since, before adjustment of the body clock to the changed local time has taken place, the normal synchrony between the endogenous and exogenous components of the circadian rhythms (see Figure 6.3) will have been lost. Some of the problems faced, particularly marked when sleep and waking activity are considered, are shown in Table 6.1.

It is this lack of synchrony between the body clock and the outside world that causes these individuals to suffer the negative subjective and objective effects that are collectively known as 'jet lag'.[1,17] The symptoms are not due to differences in climate or culture between the destination and the individual's home country. For example, they are likely to be marked for Europeans travelling to Australia, New Zealand or the west coast of America, but slight for travellers between Europe and Africa.

The symptoms of jet lag

Jet lag is an assemblage of subjective and objective symptoms. The more prominent of these are listed in Box 6.2. The wide spectrum of negative effects

Table 6.1 Some differences from living in the home time zone that will be experienced in the first days after flying across eight time zones to the east or west[1]

Local Time	Home Time Zone	After 8 Time Zones East	After 8 Time Zones West
08:00-10:00 h	Waking up	Ready to sleep	Going well
14:00-16:00 h	Going well	Only just beginning to wake up	Ready to sleep
20:00-22:00 h	Preparing to wind down	Going well	Want to be asleep
02:00-04:00 h	Sleeping well	Still going well – not sleepy	Woken up and ready to go

implies that most individuals might be affected in a way that is specifically important at a personal level. Thus, those on holiday might have their enjoyment spoiled; pilots and business people might be prone to making errors. Furthermore, athletes might be discouraged by poorer performances and lessened motivation to train hard.

Problems associated with subjective assessments of jet lag

No agreement exists at the current time for standardization of the symptoms of jet lag, or on the link that exists between the various symptoms and the assessment of jet lag itself. As a result, comparison between studies can be difficult. One more systematic approach to the problem was adopted by Spitzer et al.,[18] who obtained a high internal consistency ($\propto = 0.94$) by using the items: fatigue, difficulty concentrating, clumsiness, decreased alertness in the daytime, difficulty with memory, general weakness, dizziness, lethargy and daytime sleepiness.

Some of the classification problems that exist have been highlighted recently by ourselves.[19] First, it would be predicted that, if the symptoms shown in Box 6.2 were equally valid assessments of jet lag, then they would all be experienced most on the first day after arrival, and then decline on subsequent days with similar time courses. In one study, a group of athletes reported the severity of jet lag at five times spread regularly throughout the waking day for the first six days after flying from the UK to Australia (ten time zones to the east). In addition, they recorded regularly their fatigue, enjoyment of meals, bowel habits, mental performance and sleep. Mean daily assessments of all variables were most abnormal on the day of arrival, decreased towards normal on subsequent days, and had mostly recovered by the sixth day. However, the time-courses of recovery were different for the various symptoms. Whereas increased fatigue, decreased ability to

Box 6.2 The main symptoms of jet lag[17]

Feeling tired in the new local daytime, and yet unable to sleep at night

Feeling less able to concentrate or to motivate oneself

Decreased mental and physical performance

Increased incidence of headaches and irritability

Loss of appetite and general bowel irregularities

concentrate, and problems with some aspects of sleep (waking too early and an increased number of waking episodes during sleep) all recovered at rates similar to that of the decline of jet lag, other variables, such as decreased hunger and increased irritability, recovered with time-courses that tended to be shorter.

Whether the relationship between assessments of jet lag and its symptoms depended upon the local time in the new time zone when the assessments were made was investigated in a follow-up study.[20] On waking, jet lag might reflect the inadequacy of the previous night's sleep; during much of the daytime, it would reflect increased fatigue and decreased motivation; and, when retiring at night, jet lag would be more likely to reflect an inappropriate feeling of wakefulness at this time. The results, taken from the group of subjects who had flown from the UK to Australia, indicated that measurements of aspects of sleep disruption correlated highly with estimates of jet lag made just before retiring at night or just after rising in the morning, but not significantly with estimates of jet lag made in the middle of the daytime. Also, there was a strong correlation between estimates of jet lag made at any time of the day and fatigue measured at the same time, but not with fatigue measured at any other times of the day. For mental performance and the enjoyment of meals, the association between these variables and jet lag was weaker and applied to estimates made at wider ranges of times throughout the day.

Whatever the detailed explanation of these results, they indicate that the time at which jet lag is assessed alters the symptom(s) that the assessment reflects. It also means that assessments of the severity of jet lag made at one time of day need not indicate the severity of its symptoms at other times on the same day. This conclusion has important implications when the efficacy of methods to alleviate jet lag is investigated.

Differences between individuals in their experience of jet lag

Individuals experience the symptoms of jet lag to differing extents. In general, symptoms are worse the greater the number of time zones crossed, and on travelling eastward rather than to the west. The severity of the symptoms may also be related to menstrual cycle phase. Disturbances of this cycle, including secondary amenorrhoea, are not uncommon in air stewardesses.[21] The disturbances might arise from an interaction between melatonin secretion (which is affected by the light-dark cycle) and the oestrogens released during the menstrual cycle.

It has been suggested that the age, chronotype, sleeping habits, languor and fitness might alter their rate of adjustment to a time-zone transition.

- Age: younger subjects will have less difficulty and adjust more rapidly.
- Chronotype: those who are 'larks' (morning types) will adjust to an eastward shift more readily than 'owls' (evening types), since their body clock is phased earlier and might have a slightly shorter inherent period. The opposite should hold for time-zone transitions to the west.
- Flexibility of sleeping habits: those who are better able to adjust their times of sleeping, and who are influenced less by the conditions in which they sleep – the hardness of the mattress, for example – should be at an advantage.
- Languor: those who score highly on this measure have an inability to disregard feelings of fatigue, and experience difficulties with continuing their activities effectively if they feel fatigued. These individuals are likely to be at a disadvantage.
- Fitness: those who are physically fitter should experience fewer difficulties with adjustment.

The experimental support of these predictions is weak. In a further investigation of the subjects who flew from UK to Australia,[22] the question was posed whether any of the above acted as predictors for the amount of jet lag and its symptoms experienced after the flight. To these possible predictors were added possible effects of gender, previous experience of long-haul travel, time of arrival in Australia (the morning or late afternoon by Australian time), and direction of phase adjustment (advance or delay).

Results indicated that the scores for chronotype, flexibility of sleeping habits, languor, gender and fitness were rarely significant predictors. The only predictors that were found at all frequently were previous experience of long-haul travel, age, and time of arrival in Australia.

Those for whom such a long-haul flight was a new experience wanted to stay up rather than retire; by contrast, those who had done the flight before tended to go to bed earlier and suffered less jet lag. The finding that greater age was associated with less jet lag was the opposite of the prediction (above), but accords with the view from laboratory simulations that older subjects are better able to 'pace themselves' when dealing with the effects of sleep loss. Those subjects who arrived in Australia in the afternoon (and had left the UK in the morning) appeared to have several initial disadvantages in comparison with those who arrived early in the morning (and had left the UK in the evening). Having left the UK in the morning, they had needed to get up earlier than those who had left in the evening. Also, their first flight had been in the daytime, and they had slept significantly less on this flight than those who had left in the evening and flown through the night (about 1.5 compared with about 5.5 hours). What might have caused the observation that the afternoon arrivals suffered less jet lag? Their advantage was that they could attempt their first full sleep in a comfortable bed and during the Australian night about 30 hours after having risen from their last sleep at night in a bed in the UK. By contrast, those who had arrived in the morning, even though they had taken a nap on arrival and had slept more on the plane, did not have opportunity for a full sleep in a bed at night in Australia until about 50 hours after rising from their last sleep at night in a bed in the UK.

Jet lag was worse on days five and six after arrival in those who adjusted their body clock by a phase advance.[22] For all subjects, immediately after arrival in Australia, their temperature minimum, and time of worst performance, was at about 15:00 h by local time. For those who then adjusted by a phase delay, this time would become later, soon coinciding with the evening and a time for relaxation. By contrast, for those who adjusted by a phase advance, the time of worst performance would advance through the early afternoon and then the morning. This would account for their greater feelings of jet lag on the fifth and sixth days after arrival.

In summary, the choices of itinerary and lifestyle are more important for reducing jet lag than are personality characteristics such as chronotype or flexibility of habits. If disruptions during the working day are to be minimized, then there would also seem to be an argument for attempting to use light to promote adjustment to the new time zone by a delay rather than an advance of the body clock.

Sleep loss and decreased mental and physical performance

One of the main problems associated with jet lag is that of sleep loss.[23] After flights to the east it is getting to sleep at the new bedtime that is difficult, whereas after flights to the west the main problem tends to be premature awakening (Table 6.1). Associated with the sleep difficulties is likely to be a risk of performance decrement. It has been suggested that jet lag might be associated with errors or accidents.[24,25] A report by Samel et al.[26] supports this view. Pilots on long-haul flights to the east and west were studied. Particularly with flights to the east at night, pilot fatigue increased during the flight to values that could be assumed to be associated with performance decrement. Moreover, EEG recordings indicated a mean occurrence of up to five 'microevents' per hour during the 'cruise phase of the flight. (A microevent was defined as an 8-second period where brain α–activity rose above a certain threshold; it is also known as a 'microsleep'.)

The widespread negative effects of sleep loss upon mood have been found in field studies of military and civilian subjects, and in laboratory studies. It has been argued that such deterioration can adversely affect group activities and motivation, and is therefore likely to be important for athletes in training. By contrast, muscle strength is generally found to be resistant to any deterioration after sleep loss, as has physical activity – there being no fall in

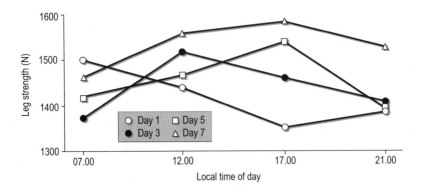

Figure 6.4 Change in local timing of leg strength (Newtons) on Days 1, 3 and 7 after a westward flight across 5 time zones[1]

self-chosen work-rate or rise in perceived exertion and heart rate in the sleep-deprivation condition. Studies indicate a deterioration in performance in 'marathon' exhibitions where sleep is lost over several consecutive nights.[27] In these, however, activity is continuous and has to be sustained; as with mental performance, deterioration seems to be considerably less when short rests are interposed.

For competitors at the international level, most results indicate a poorer performance (of activities involving complex mental activity rather than physical strength), a feeling of lethargy and a general loss of motivation after time-zone transitions.[1] The problems due to jet lag are twofold. First, maximum performance might be lessened if it does not coincide with the individual's circadian peak; second, serious training might be jeopardised due to inappropriate times of training as well as increased fatigue and subsequent negative effects on mood and physical and mental performance. An increased time taken for both a sprint and a middle-distance race after an eastward flight crossing six time zones has been shown. Also, British Rugby League players who travelled to Australia showed a disturbance in their circadian rhythm in grip strength, which normally peaks in the evening. Only by the fourth day were strength values in the evening higher than the morning scores, and it took two to three more days for the normal circadian rhythm to restore itself. Similarly, leg strength showed a circadian rhythm disturbance in a group of athletes on the first day after a westward transition across five time zones (Figure 6.4); the time of peak strength did not shift to its normal value of about 17:00 h until about the fifth day post-flight.

Training programmes should take into account that some of the new daytime will correspond to night in the time zone just left and that the athlete or games player will also be suffering from the effects of sleep loss. Restricted training schedules and reduced levels of achievement should be expected by both the coach and the athlete or player during this time of adjustment to the new time zone.

ADVICE REGARDING JET LAG

Brief stays (three days or less) in the new time zone

If the stay in the new time zone is going to be for a few days only, then there will not be enough time for the body clock to adjust. In these cases, many travellers, including aircrew, continue to live as much as possible on home time. This means that, after a flight to the east, important activities should be undertaken in the afternoon or evening by local time in the new environment (coincident with daytime on home time), and the morning should be left free for relaxation or sleep (coincident with night on home time). If the flight is to the west, then important activities should be arranged for the morning, the afternoon and evening being for relaxation and sleep.

Longer stays in the new time zone

If the stay in the new time zone is for several days, then adjustment of the body clock, and adherence to local time, should be attempted. The following advice is the best currently available for minimizing disruptions to sleep and performance in the new time zone. It is important to realise that it applies particularly to the first day or so in the new time zone, that some of it applies as soon as the home time zone has been left behind, and some applies even when plans for the flights are being made.

Before travel

Attempts to find the most convenient travel schedules are encouraged. Any recommendation should bear in mind the evidence that jet lag is less if the total time that elapses between the last proper sleep in the country being left and the first proper sleep in the destination country is as short as possible. Also, itineraries involving a stopover *en route* of a day or so are worth considering. This is because it has been found in jet lag simulation studies that dividing the total time-zone transition into more than one sector (for example a 10-hour shift into shifts of 7 hours and 3 hours) resulted in a decrease in the severity of jet lag.[28] Practically, however, the advantages of such a stopover should be weighed against increased cost and the doubling of any stresses due to baggage transportation, passport controls and searching for accommodation.

During travel

Advice regarding the dry cabin atmosphere and the cramped conditions of travel applies here. There is the additional issue of deciding whether or not to sleep.

If adjustment of the body clock is being attempted, then naps and sleep should be avoided unless they coincide with night at the *destination* or unless individuals have been chronically deprived of sleep during transit. If it is daytime at the destination, therefore, the traveller should attempt to stay awake by reading, playing cards or investigating the in-flight entertainment, for example. A good piece of advice is to realise that, as soon as the plane has been boarded, 'home time' has been left behind and should be erased from the traveller's mind; instead, it is the time at the destination or stop-over point that now determines when things should be done. Changing one's watch immediately on boarding the plane should help in achieving this attitude of mind.

One possibility is to use sleeping pills to promote sleep.[29] Some travellers have used minor tranquillizers, such as temazepam and zolpiden, and other members of the diazepine group, in order to be refreshed for immediate activities on arrival. However, even if the drug does help a person get to sleep, it does not guarantee a prolonged period of sleep, nor has it always been satisfactorily tested for subsequent residual effects on mental or physical performance. It is also important to realise that sleeping pills might be counter-productive if given at the incorrect time. A prolonged sleep at the time an individual feels drowsy, presumably when he or she would have been asleep in the time zone just left, anchors the rhythms to this time zone and so operates against adjustment to the new time zone.

After travel

General lifestyle

In general, the advice is to adjust the sleep-wake schedule and mealtimes as rapidly and fully as possible to those in the destination. This might include sight-seeing in the first day or so after arrival, but there are potential problems with this as regards light exposure, problems that will be considered later.

For athletes, training sessions should not be all-out efforts in the first days after arrival. Skills requiring fine co-ordination are likely to be impaired and this might lead to accidents or injuries if, for example, games players conduct sessions with the ball too strenuously. Where a series of tournament engagements is scheduled, it is useful to have at least one friendly match during the initial period – that is, before the end of the first week – in the overseas country. Subject to these caveats, exercise for athletes is recommended since it helps them psychologically in their preparations for competition.

Until the body clock is adjusted to the new local time, there will be a window of time during the day when the period of high arousal associated with the time zone just left overlaps with the arousal high point at the new local time. This window can be estimated in advance and should be utilized for timing of training practices in the first few days at the destination.

General lifestyle and exposure to light can be used to promote adjustment of the body clock by a delay or an advance. For example,[30] when the arrival time of a group of athletes travelling eastward from the UK to Oceania (Australia and New Zealand) was in the early morning, they were allowed to sleep on arrival until midday, and then allowed outdoors in the afternoon. When the arrival time was in the late afternoon, they were encouraged to be outdoors rather than to sleep. In both cases, this regimen of exposure to natural daylight in the later part of the day would promote a phase advance of the body clock. Conversely, athletes travelling westward to Oceania from the UK have utilized a behavioural regimen that favoured a phase delay of the body clock.

Promoting sleep and alertness
Drugs have been used to promote sleep in the new time zones, important amongst which are the benzodiazepines.[29,31,32] However, Reilly et al.[33] found no beneficial effects of temazepam in Olympic athletes travelling from London to Florida (five time zones to the west). In such a case, it seems that disembarkation in the late evening local time might help in getting to sleep following a westward flight, thereby diminishing any potential effect of the drug.

In practice, the problem is often one of making sure that travellers are fully awake and alert after waking up the next day. Most of the benzodiazepines are associated with residual effects on alertness and psychomotor performance. Temazepam may be less problematic in this respect, since its half-life is only 2-8 hours compared to diazepam's 24-48 hours. Recently, interest has been shown in zolpiden, which has a short half-life and affects short-term memory less than other drugs of this group. In their review, Stone and Turner[32] concluded that 'advice on the use of hypnotics requires further clarification' but they acknowledged that the general usefulness of such drugs was beyond doubt.

Promoting alertness is another approach to the difficulties of jet lag, but this option has been investigated less. Akerstedt and Ficca[34] considered amphetamines, caffeine, the α_1–adrenoceptor agonist modafinil, and pemoline, a drug with dopamine-like properties. These drugs have been used to sustain alertness and performance at mental tasks during extended periods without sleep and for treating narcolepsy. Although they improve mental performance at several tasks, they also reduce the ability to initiate and sustain sleep, an effect which might be counterproductive. There is evidence that amphetamines can compromise decision-making and psychomotor performance, and there is potential for drug abuse. Caffeine has been linked to heart arrhythmias and the development of drug dependence. Pemoline and modafinil have less deleterious effects upon complex mental tasks and far less potential for drug abuse. Even so, further work is required before any firm recommendation can be made regarding the use of drugs to promote alertness after time-zone transitions. For athletes, the use of such drugs may be out of the question as they are included in the list of banned substqances published by the International Olympic Committee.

Clock-shifting – general principles
The main advice is to aim at promoting adjustment of the body clock to the new time zone. Several methods have been suggested, differing in their practicality, the scientific evidence in support of them, and in potential side-

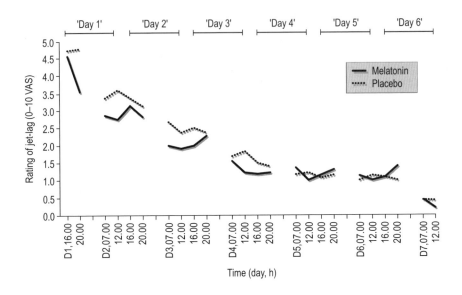

Figure 6.5 Mean (± SD) jet lag (measured on a Visual Analogue Scale, VAS) in control group (placebo, N=17) and experimental group (melatonin, N=14) during the first days after a flight from UK to Australia[39]

effects. They include nutritional, environmental and behavioural measures. In effect, they often amount to strengthening the zeitgebers in the new time zone.

Redfern[31] stressed the unlikelihood of chronopharmacologists developing a panacea-like 'jet lag pill', since the circadian system was so complicated, with multiple input and output signals to and from the body clock. Dawson and Armstrong[35] listed many classes of drugs that had the capacity to modify the circadian system ('chronobiotics'); however, many of these have been tested only on animals. Attention here will be directed mainly to the two methods that seem to be most effective: melatonin and bright light.

When attempting to promote adjustment of the body clock, it is essential to understand that this process can take place either by advancing or delaying it, and that each alternative requires a different timing of treatment. For time-zone transitions of up to eight hours to the east, a phase advance of the body clock should be promoted, and for time-zone transitions to the west, a phase delay. For journeys to the east through nine or more time zones, the position is more complex, since adjustment could be by advance or delay.[36] In practice, delaying the phase of the body clock is sometimes easier, because this way the time of minimum temperature and poorest performance delays into the evening rather than advances into the morning.

Clock shifting – the use of melatonin

In normal circumstances, melatonin from the pineal gland is secreted into the bloodstream between about 21:00 and 07:00 h, and can be regarded as a 'dark pulse' or 'internal zeitgeber' for the body clock.[7] Melatonin capsules taken in the evening by local time in the new time zone reduce the symptoms of jet lag, the effect having been confirmed in both genders, after flights in either direction, and at whatever time the flight takes place. Recent reviews have appeared.[37,38]

Not all studies have shown that melatonin significantly ameliorates the problems associated with time-zone transitions. Studies by Spitzer et al.,[18] and by Edwards et al.[39] involved shifts eastwards across six or ten time zones (Figure 6.5). Exactly why these studies should have produced negative results is unclear, but several possibilities exist. First, in the study of Edwards et al.,[39] the subjects were sports scientists, and elite sportspersons preparing for the Olympic Games. All were extremely highly motivated, and determined not to be adversely affected by any negative effects associated with travel. Such a degree of motivation might be an inappropriate background against which to measure the effect of a treatment for the debilitating effects of jet lag. Second, in both studies, as in most others, the subjects' exposure to natural lighting was not controlled. There is evidence that melatonin administration cannot counteract phase shifts produced by light given at the same time. These findings indicate that exposure to the light-dark cycle, particularly to natural lighting, might have overwhelmed any effects due to melatonin.

In some studies, melatonin ingestion has been found to exert wider beneficial effects than improving sleep.[8] Other benefits documented have included acceleration of adjustment of core temperature and urinary variables in a laboratory simulation; a decrease in errors in a vigilance task in a field study upon aircrew; improvment in mental performance in a simulation study; acceleration of adjustment of the melatonin rhythm in a field study; acceleration of adjustment of cortisol and melatonin rhythms in field study conditions; maintainance of some aspects of physical performance in the field; and acceleration of adjustment of blood pressure in a single male flying from Milan to Houston. In other studies, by contrast, melatonin has been found not to change core temperature or mental performance in the same way as it affected sleep and assessments of jet lag. Nevertheless, there is increasing evidence to support its use in the short term, with little indication of serious side effects. An individual is recommended to take medical advice before taking melatonin for the first time, and not to do so if young, pregnant or lactating, or if an important event is to take place immediately after arrival in the new time zone.[40]

There remain some caveats to the general advisability of taking melatonin:[17,40]

- Jet lag, as defined in these studies, has concentrated on subjective symptoms and on the ability to sleep; it is not clear that there are always comparable improvements in mental and physical performance. Clearly, for aircrew, athletes and businesspersons, for example, it would be disadvantageous if residual effects were present. However, in a study performed on subjects who were living normally and had not undergone a time-zone transition, melatonin capsules were ingested in the early

Table 6.2 The use of bright light to adjust the body clock after time-zone transitions[17]

	Bad local times for exposure to bright light	Good local times for exposure to bright light
Time zones to the west		
4 h	01:00-07:00[a]	17:00-23:00[b]
8 h	21:00-03:00[a]	13:00-19:00[b]
12 h	17:00-23:00[a]	09:00-15:00[b]
16 h	13:00-19:00[a]	05:00-11:00[b]
Time zones to the east		
4 h	01:00-07:00[b]	09:00-15:00[a]
8 h	05:00-11:00[b]	13:00-19:00[a]
10-12 h	Treat these as 14-12 h to the west, respectively[c]	

Notes:
[a] this will advance the body clock
[b] this will delay the body clock
[c] this is because the body clock adjusts to large delays more easily than to large advances

evening.[41] The following morning, the subjects did not report any fall in alertness, mental performance or physical performance compared with the occasion when they took a placebo.

- The mechanism(s) by which melatonin acts are uncertain. There are two obvious possibilities: it might act as a hypnotic or as a chronobiotic. The hypnotic effect is believed to be related to the fall of core temperature that results from the vasodilatation that melatonin causes, MT_2 receptors being implicated in this change in blood flow.[8] The chronobiotic action stems from the demonstration of a phase response curve (PRC) to melatonin.[13] This indicates that, in entrained subjects living normally, phase advances are produced by administration between 13:00 and 01:00 h (with peak advances at about 19:00 h) and delays by administration between 01:00 and 13:00 h (with peak delays at about 07:00 h).

- Before melatonin can be recommended for extended use, in aircrew for example, it is necessary to establish that there are no adverse long-term effects. It has been argued that such effects might exist, but they have not been tested, and the lack of data pertaining to this issue has been stressed.[42] Further work is urgently required, as has been stated recently.[43]

In summary, more information is required before melatonin can be recommended unreservedly. In those cases where an individual has taken melatonin before, and has found it to be beneficial and with no adverse side-effects, there is currently no evidence against using it again. Nevertheless, medical advice should be sought.

Clock shifting – the use of bright light The effectiveness of natural light in adjusting the body clock in humans has already been described, and tables (Table 6.2) and computer programmes exist which advise travellers on when to attempt exposure to, or avoidance of, bright light. They are based on the observations that bright light in the morning (05:00-11:00 h) on body time advances the clock and bright light in the evening (22:00-04:00 h) on body time delays it.[9,10] As a supplement to this treatment there are also times when light should be avoided (those times which produce a shift of the body clock in the direction opposite to that desired). On subsequent days, when partial adjustment of the body clock has occurred, the individual is advised to alter the timings of light exposure and avoidance towards the local light-dark cycle by one hour per day. In this way, the traveller's exposure to light gradually becomes synchronized with that of the locals.

A problem exists, however, in that the times of light-seeking and light-avoidance may not concur with the natural alternation between daytime and night. Avoiding bright light, by staying indoors and/or wearing dark glasses, is comparatively easy; seeking bright light is more of a problem. 'Light boxes', which mimic sunlight in spectral emission and brightness, are available, but they are normally cumbersome. Visors, portable light sources with their own power, are now becoming available. However, the demonstration that light of an intensity found domestically can determine the phasing of the body clock might obviate the need for such visors.

Adjusting as fully as possible to the lifestyle and habits in the new zone, and so being exposed to the new natural light-dark cycle, would seem intuitively to be the best remedy; this intuition is borne out by the example of a westward flight through eight time zones. To delay the clock requires exposure to bright light at 21:00-03:00 h body time and avoidance of it at 05:00-11:00 h body time on the first day. By new local time (see Table 6.2), this becomes equal to 13:00-19:00 h for bright light exposure and 21:00-03:00 h for bright light avoidance, staying indoors in dim light. (On the second day in the new time zone, light exposure at 14:00-20:00 h and light avoidance at 22:00-04:00 h are required, and so on.) Exposure to the new local day-night cycle – by getting 'out and about' and mixing with the local people – would provide this. For light after a westward shift, there is therefore no need to deviate from the timing of natural light.

Consider, instead, a flight to the east through eight time zones, when a phase advance of the body clock is advised. This (see Table 6.2) requires bright light exposure at 05:00-11:00 h *body time* (13:00-19:00 h local time) and dim light (light avoidance) at 21:00-03:00 h *body time* (05:00-11:00 h local time). (On subsequent days, light exposure and avoidance times can become earlier by about 1-2 hours per day until they coincide with natural lighting.) It can be seen from this requirement that morning light for the first day or so would be unhelpful and tend to make the clock adjust in the wrong direction – though afternoon and evening light are fine. The advice about getting 'out and about' and mixing with local people needs to be modified in this case, therefore, as it would be better to spend the morning indoors. This is one explanation of why adjustment to phase advances is more difficult to achieve than is adjustment to phase delays.

For flights to the east crossing more than nine time zones, a choice exists with regard to whether one uses light exposure and avoidance to delay or to advance the body clock.[36] For example, after a flight to the east coast of Australia from the UK (an eastward flight through ten time zones), Table 6.4 can be used either by treating the flight as an eastward one across ten time zones or as a westward one through fourteen time zones. The choice is up to individuals, but they must stick to one regimen throughout the process of adjustment, of course. They would be advised to select the light exposure-avoidance regimen that better fits in with their plans. For example, on arrival, the time of minimum body temperature, poorest performance and maximum fatigue will be at about 15:00 h local time. If a phase advance of the body clock is being attempted, then arrival in daylight in the morning by local time (which will be before the temperature minimum) will promote a phase delay of the body clock – unless the light is avoided and dark sunglasses are worn until the shelter of a dimly-lit hotel room is reached. By contrast, arrival in daylight in the local late afternoon or early evening (which will be after the temperature minimum) will promote a phase advance of the body clock, unless the bright light is avoided. Moreover, if a phase advance of the body clock is being attempted, then the times of minimum body temperature, poorest performance and maximum fatigue will advance through the afternoon and morning on subsequent days. The effects of jet lag will be noticed more in this case than in the case where a delay is attempted, since, with a delay, the time of poorest performance will progress through the afternoon and evening, and fit in better with relaxing at these times.[22]

Clock shifting – diet and exercise Other means to promote adjustment of the body clock have been proposed for humans, such as feeding/fasting and physical activity/inactivity cycles. The current evidence for them is unconvincing.

The 'feeding hypothesis'[44] proposes that a high protein breakfast raises plasma tyrosine levels and that this promotes the synthesis and release of the neurotransmitters noradrenaline and dopamine, so activating the arousal system of the body. Similarly, a high carbohydrate evening meal will raise plasma tryptophan levels and this promotes the synthesis and release of serotonin, a major neurotransmitter of the raphé nucleus (important in sleep regulation) and a precursor of melatonin.

Evidence favouring the feeding hypothesis is not strong. First, it was tested upon a group of military personnel undergoing an eastward time-zone transition of nine hours, but only small improvements in sleep and performance at mental tasks were observed, and the control and

> **Box 6.3 Checklist for dealing with jet lag**[16]
>
> 1. Check if the journey is across sufficient time zones for jet lag to be a problem. If it is not, then it is necessary only to refer to advice on overcoming travel fatigue (Box 6.1).
> 2. If jet lag is likely, then consider if the stay is too short for adjustment of the body clock to take place (a stay of less than 3 days). If it is too short, then remain on home time, and attempt to arrange sleep and activities to coincide with this as much as possible.
> 3. If the stay is not too short (3 days or more) and it is wished to promote adjustment, then consider ways of reducing jet lag. Advice relates to:
>   Before the flight;
>   During the flight;
>   After the flight.
>   The most important advice relates to after the flight.
> 4. Advice for promoting adjustment concentrates on:
>   Sleep and melatonin;
>   Exposure to, and avoidance of, bright light (Table 6.2);
>   Behavioural factors.

experimental groups appear to have been treated slightly differently.[45] Second, experiments upon rodents do not support the basic requirement of the hypothesis that plasma levels of tyrosine or tryptophan are rate-limiting stages for neurotransmitter release.[44]

If hamsters[46] act as a model for humans, then physical activity should promote adjustment of the body clock, although it might not be the activity *per se* but rather the CNS arousal that is produced by it that is effective. Results with humans have not yet proved convincing evidence for the phase-shifting effects of exercise (see Edwards et al.[47]), though whether this indicates that such a mechanism is inoperative in humans because the amount of activity needs to be greater, or because subjects must be more 'excited' by exercise, is unclear. Nevertheless, to combine appropriately-timed exposure to bright light with activity outdoors, and bright light avoidance with staying indoors and relaxing, would seem worth considering.

A check list for dealing with jet lag is given in Box 6.3. Estimates of how long jet lag will last, if the ameliorative measures are adhered to, are given in Table 6.3.

SLOW TRANSITIONS ACROSS TIME ZONES

Whilst journeys across and between continents generally involve rapid flights, slower means of travel, by ocean liner or car, for example, are still used. In such cases, the time-zone transitions are accomplished much more slowly. At the equator, one time zone is approximately 1000 miles (1600 km), which means that the traveller will cross less than one time zone per day. This

Table 6.3 Estimates of how long jet lag will last[16]

Westward flights		Eastward flights	
Time zones crossed	Days to adjust	Time zones crossed	Days to adjust
0-3	0 [a]	0-2	0 [a]
4-6	1-3	3-5	1-5
7-9	2-5	6-8	3-7
10-12	3-6	9-11	4-9

[a] Day of rest recommended to recover from travel fatigue

should produce very little inconvenience, the body clock normally being advanced by 30 minutes per day in subjects adjusted to the 24-hour solar day. Its effects would be comparable with those produced when local time is adjusted by one hour in the switches from winter to summer time. Cruising from Europe to America, for example, would enable the traveller to go to bed and get up about one hour later each day, something that many people choose to do at the weekends.

The problems are very different for those who sail or row across oceans. In these cases, the problem is generally one of getting enough sleep in an environment in which continuous alertness and effort are required. Laboratory studies indicate that sleep loss of as little as two hours can lead to a deterioration in some aspects of mental performance and, in general, the decrement in mental performance appears to increase with the total amount of sleep lost.[48-50] The performance decrement does not show itself as an equal decline at all times and in all circumstances; it can be worse for repetitive tasks and when the core temperature is near its trough. 'Micro-sleeps' might occur, during which subjects appear to be awake but are unaware of what is happening around them. Physical activities appear to be more resilient with regard to the negative effects of sleep loss, but general mood and motivation to work are likely to be affected adversely. It has been shown that periods of sleep of as little as 1-2 hours per 24 hours are able to ameliorate some of the effects of sleep deprivation, and that longer sleeps (whilst still not long enough to prevent symptoms of sleep loss entirely) are even more effective.

There has been a tendency for those individuals who face the prospect of prolonged effort and potential sleep loss to change from the normal pattern of 8 hours sleep and 16 hours of waking each 24 hours. Instead, the practices of living shorter 'days' and 'power napping' have developed – for example, dividing the 24 hours into two 'days' of 4 hours sleep and 8 hours waking, or four 'days' of 2 hours sleep and 4 hours waking. These retain the normal balance between time awake and asleep, and have the advantage that the periods of activity – which causes fatigue – and the periods when the individual is asleep – and not contributing to the overall effort of sailing or rowing – are both decreased.

Laboratory studies have shown that such schemes do not result in any obvious adverse side-effects when implemented for several days. The evidence indicates that sleep and its various stages continue to be taken, and that fatigue builds up less during the shorter periods of activity. There does, however, appear to be a limit to how short the 'day' can be, this being determined by the abilities to take recuperative, 'deep' (slow wave) sleep and to overcome the effects of 'sleep inertia' immediately after waking.[49-51] Opportunities for sleep that are much shorter than two hours limit this ability.

OVERVIEW

The traveller faces several problems that can decrease the sense of well-being and even impair mental and physical performance. These range from acute effects for the long-distance traveller who crosses few time zones, through to the effects of jet lag, that last a week or so if several time zones are crossed, to the longer-lasting effects in those who crew yachts or row boats for long distances.

The science of chronobiology enables an understanding of the kinds of problem that will be associated with such changes, these often centring on sleep loss and its effects. The knowledge so obtained can then form the rational basis for advice to the traveller. The most common problem is that of jet lag. Implementing the advice will not remove jet lag, but it will reduce it towards a minimum, a minimum that will depend upon the individual.

References

1. Reilly T, Atkinson G, Waterhouse J. Biological rhythms and exercise. Oxford: Oxford University Press, 1997
2. Redfern P, Waterhouse J, Minors D. Circadian rhythms: principles and measurement. Pharmacol Therapeut 1991; 49:311-327
3. Atkinson G, Coldwells A, Reilly T et al. Circadian rhythmicity in self-chosen work-rate. In: Chronobiology and chronomedicine: basic research and applications. Gutenbrunner C, Hildebrandt G, Moog R (eds). Frankfurt: Lang-Verlag, 1993:478-484
4. Minors D, Waterhouse J. Circadian rhythms and the human. Bristol: John Wright, 1981
5. Moore R. Organisation of the mammalian circadian system. In: Circadian clocks and their adjustment. Chadwick D, Ackrill K (eds). Ciba Foundation Symposium, 183. Chichester: Wiley, 1995:88-106
6. Clayton J, Kyriacou C, Reppert S. Keeping time with the human genome. Nature 2001; 409:829-831
7. Arendt J. The pineal. In: Biological rhythms in clinical and laboratory medicine. Touitou Y, Haus E (eds). Berlin: Springer-Verlag, 1992:348-362
8. Atkinson G, Drust B, Reilly T et al. The relevance of melatonin to sports medicine and science. Sports Medicine 2003 ; 33:809-831
9. Czeisler C, Kronauer R, Duffy J et al. Bright light induction of strong (Type 0) resetting of the human circadian pacemaker. Science 1989; 244:1328-1333

10. Minors D, Waterhouse J, Wirz-Justice A. A human phase-response curve to light. Neurosci Lett 1991; 133:36-40
11. Boivin D, Duffy J, Kronauer R et al. Dose-response relationship for resetting of human circadian clock by light. Nature 1996; 379:540-542
12. Waterhouse J, Minors D, Folkard S et al. Light of domestic intensity produces phase shifts of the circadian oscillator in humans. Neurosci Lett 1998; 245:97-100
13. Lewy A, Bauer V, Ahmed S et al. The human phase response curve (PRC) to melatonin is about 12 hours out of phase with the PRC to light. Chronobiol Int 1998, 15:71-83
14. Lewy A, Sack R. The role of melatonin and light in the human circadian system. Prog in Brain Res 1996; 111:205-216
15. Miyamoto Y, Sancar A. Vitamin B_2-based blue-light photoreceptors in the retinohypothalamic tract as the photoactive pigments for setting the circadian clock in mammals. Proc Nat Acad Sci 1998; 95:6097-6102
16. Waterhouse JM, Minors DS, Waterhouse ME et al. Keeping in time with your body clock. Oxford: Oxford University Press, 2002
17. Waterhouse J, Reilly T, Atkinson G. Jet-lag. Lancet 1997; 350:1611-1615
18. Spitzer R, Terman M, Williams J et al. Jet lag: clinical features, validation of a new syndrome-specific scale, and lack of response to melatonin in a randomised, double-blind trial. Amer J Psychiatry 1999; 156:1392-1396
19. Waterhouse J, Edwards B, Nevill A et al. Do subjective symptoms predict our perception of jet lag? Ergonomics 2000; 43:1514-1527
20. Waterhouse J, Nevill A, Edwards B et al. The relationship between assessments of jet lag and some of its symptoms. Chronobiol Int 2003 ; 20:1061-1073
21. Suvanto S, Härma M, Ilmarinen J et al. Effects of 10 h time zone changes on female flight attendants' circadian rhythms of body temperature, alertness and visual search. Ergonomics 1993; 36:613-625
22. Waterhouse J, Edwards B, Nevill A et al. Identifying some determinants of 'jet lag' and its symptoms: a study of athletes and other travellers. Brit J Sports Med 2002; 36:54-60
23. Gander P, Nguyen D, Rosekind M et al. Age, circadian rhythms and sleep loss in flight crews. Aviat Space Environ Med 1993; 64:189-195
24. Akerstedt T. Work hours, sleepiness and accidents. J Sleep Res 1995; 4 (Suppl 2):1-3
25. Dinges D. An overview of sleepiness and accidents. J Sleep Res 1995; 4 (Suppl 2):4-14
26. Samel A, Wegmann H, Vejvoda M. Jet lag and sleepiness in aircrew. J Sleep Res 1995; 4 (Suppl 2): 30-36
27. Reilly T. Circadian rhythms. In: Oxford textbook of sports medicine. Harries M, Williams C, Stanish W et al (eds). New York: Oxford University Press, 1994:238-254
28. Tsai T, Okumura M, Yamasaki M et al. Simulation of jet lag following a trip with stopovers by intermittent schedule shifts. J Interdisc Cycle Res 1988; 19:89-96
29. Atkinson G, Reilly T, Waterhouse J et al. Pharmacology and the travelling athlete. In: The clinical pharmacology of sports and exercise. Reilly T, Orme M (eds). Amsterdam: Elsevier, 1997:293-301
30. Reilly T, Mellor S. Jet-lag in student Rugby League players following a near maximal time-zone shift. In: Science and football. Reilly T, Lees A, Davids K et al (eds). London: Spon, 1988:249-256
31. Redfern P. 'Jet-lag': strategies for prevention and cure. Hum Psychopharmacol 1989; 4:159-168
32. Stone B, Turner C. Promoting sleep in shiftworkers and intercontinental travellers. Chronobiol Int 1997; 14:133-143
33. Reilly T, Atkinson G, Budgett R. Effects of temazepam on physiological and performance variables following a westerly flight across five time zones. J Sports Sci 1997; 15:62

34. Akerstedt T, Ficca G. Alertness-enhancing drugs as a countermeasure to fatigue in irregular work hours. Chronobiol Int 1997; 14:145-158
35. Dawson D, Armstrong S. Chronobiotics – drugs that shift rhythms. Pharmacol Ther 1996; 69:15-36
36. Gundel A, Wegmann H. Transition between advance and delay responses to eastbound transmeridian flights. Chronobiol Int 1989; 6:147-156
37. Haimov I, Arendt J. The prevention and treatment of jet lag. Sleep Med Rev 1999; 3:229-240
38. Herxheimer A, Petrie K. Melatonin for the prevention and treatment of jet lag (Cochrane Review). In: The Cochrane Library, Issue 4. Oxford: Update Software, 2002
39. Edwards B, Atkinson G, Waterhouse J et al. Use of melatonin in recovery from jet-lag following an eastward flight across 10 time-zones. Ergonomics 2000; 43:1501-1513
40. Reilly T, Maughan R, Budgett R. Melatonin: a position statement of the British Olympic Association. Brit J Sports Med 1998; 32:99-100
41. Atkinson G, Buckley P, Edwards B et al. Are there hangover-effects on physical performance when melatonin is ingested by athletes before nocturnal sleep? Int J Sports Med 2001; 22:232-234
42. Guardiola-Lemaitre B. Toxicology of melatonin. J Biol Rhythms 1997; 12:697-706
43. Herxheimer A, Waterhouse J. Editorial: the prevention and treatment of jet lag. BMJ 2003; 326:296-297
44. Leathwood P. Circadian rhythms of plasma amino acids, brain neurotransmitters and behaviour. In: Biological rhythms in clinical practice. Arendt J, Minors D, Waterhouse J (eds). Guildford: Butterworths, 1989:136-159
45. Graeber R. Alterations in performance following rapid transmeridian flight. In: Rhythmic aspects of behaviour. Brown F, Graeber R (eds). New Jersey: Lawrence Erlbaum, 1982:173-212
46. Redlin U, Mrosovsky N. Exercise and human circadian rhythms: what we know and what we need to know. Chronobiol Int 1997; 14:221-229
47. Edwards B, Waterhouse J, Atkinson G et al. Exercise does not necessarily influence the phase of the circadian rhythm in temperature in humans. J Sports Sci 2002; 20:725-732
48. Graeber R. Jet lag and sleep disruption. In: Principles and practice of sleep medicine. Krugger M, Roth T, Dement C (eds). Philadelphia/London: WB Saunders, 1989:324-331
49. Dinges D. Adult napping and its effect on ability to function. In: Why we nap. Stampi C (ed). Boston: Birkhauser, 1992:118-134
50. Naitoh P, Kelly T, Babkoff H. Sleep inertia: best time not to wake up? Chronobiol Int 1993; 10:109-118
51. Naitoh P. Minimal sleep to maintain performance: the search for sleep quantum in sustained operations. In: Why we nap. Stampi C (ed). Boston: Birkhauser, 1992:199-216

Chapter 7

The effects of space flight

CHAPTER CONTENTS

Introduction 117
The physics of the effects of gravity
  and acceleration forces upon
  columns of fluid 119

Increased G-forces 122
Physiological effects of weightlessness
  127
Overview 141

INTRODUCTION

For the general public, the 'Space Age' opened in 1957, with the launching of Sputnik I, a Russian satellite which orbited the Earth about once every 90 minutes. Later in that year, a dog, Laika, became the first living animal to orbit the Earth, and this was followed in 1961 by the first orbit of the Earth by a human, the Russian, Yuri Gagarin. The Americans joined what became known as the 'Space Race', and landed two men on the moon, Neil Armstrong and Buzz Aldrin, in 1969. Armstrong's words on stepping onto the moon – 'It's one small step for man, one giant leap for mankind' – have passed into folklore.

Even though unmanned probes have flown past, orbited and landed safely upon the moon and planets in the solar system, it continues to be the presence of humans in space that excites the imagination – consider the flight of Apollo 13 in 1970 when the mission had to be aborted, and the astronauts' lives were in jeopardy, for example.

More recent years have seen the development of space stations, which permanently orbit the Earth and allow humans to remain in them for extended periods of time. Establishing the response of humans to extended periods of time in space is a necessary prerequisite for manned missions to other planets, where the return journeys will take years. Initially, the space stations were developed for exclusive use by the Russians (Salyut I, 1971) or Americans (Skylab, 1973) but, in 1975, co-operation was initiated by the

What's involved:

You will undergo the most intense medical examination of your life. Over the course of ten days, you will be given a variety of detailed medical tests at Moscow's Institute of Medical and Biological Problems.

The IMBP was established in 1963 and is the Institute responsible for all aspects of medical and biological support for humans in space, from selection of cosmonauts to in flight support and rehabilitation. You will receive all the same tests given to IMBP's "normal" clients – Russia's top test pilots and scientists hoping to be accepted into Russia's Space Program.

As part of your cosmonaut qualification course, you'll receive an introduction to space training which includes the following:

- Hypobaric altitude chamber testing
- Hands on training on Star City's many simulators
- Orlan space suit training
- Centrifuge training
- Vestibular training
- Personal zero-gravity flight
- Instruction and sample space mission in the hydrolab *
- Flight to the edge of space in a Russian MiG-25

* In the event medical tests show you are ineligible for hydrolab training, we will substitute a supersonic flight in a MiG-29 jet fighter.

Figure 7.1 Information about tourist flights to space (from www.incredible-adventures.com)

docking of the three-man Apollo spacecraft with a two-man Soyuz craft. The year 1981 saw the first flight of a re-usable shuttle craft, which is a more economical way of exchanging crew and materials between the Earth and space stations, and in 1983 the first European Skylab was launched. The first permanently manned space station, Mir, was launched by the Russians in 1986, and continued to produce scientifically useful results for about 15 years. In recent years, a new permanent space station has been in orbit, manned by astronauts from several countries, though mainly the USA, the CIS (Confederation of Independent States, formerly known as the Union of Soviet Socialist Republics, USSR) and Europe.

The early astronauts were mainly testpilots and others with similar skills, but later missions have included scientists and even members of the general public; the era of 'space tourism' has begun, provided that the individual can afford the tour – currently, a few million dollars! An Internet search easily reveals sites that give information about applying for such tours, though the selection procedures are necessarily extremely rigorous and time-consuming (Figure 7.1).

Assuming that an individual is in perfect health, what are the demands of space flight, and how well is a human able to adjust to these needs?

THE PHYSICS OF THE EFFECTS OF GRAVITY AND ACCELERATION FORCES UPON COLUMNS OF FLUID

When a person stands upright from the lying position, there is a transient fall in blood pressure. If the movement is carried out too quickly, there is a risk of transient dizziness (orthostatic hypotension). These changes are due to pooling of blood in the legs and the decreased venous return that this produces. In turn, cardiac output and blood pressure fall transiently. Normally, these changes are quickly corrected by the baroreceptor reflexes.

The blood vessels are filled with blood and the pressure measured at any point in the circuit is determined not only by the pumping activity of the heart but also by the pressure exerted by the column of fluid lying between the measurement point and some reference point. In cardiovascular studies, this reference point is often taken as the level of the heart. The pressure, P, exerted by the column of blood is given by the equation:

$$P = \pm h.p.G$$

Pressure can be conveniently expressed as cm H_2O, if h, the vertical distance between the measurement point and the heart, is expressed in cm; p, the density of the fluid, is expressed in g/cm^3 (in practice, for blood it is taken to be 1.0); and G, the acceleration due to gravity, is expressed as a multiple of the normal gravitational force (and so is described as 1-G in stationary subjects on Earth). If the measurement point is above the reference point, then the pressure will be lower; if it is below it, then the pressure is higher.

In a subject lying down at rest, the legs are at about the same height as the heart, and so there is no effect of pressure due to the column of blood since h is zero. After standing up, however, the legs are below the level of the heart, and so the pressure inside the leg vessels increases by h cm H_2O, where h is the distance between the point of measurement and the heart. The pressure outside the vessels does not change, because the pressure in the extravascular tissue is equal to the (unchanged) pressure in the surrounding environment. There is, therefore, an increase in transmural pressure across all blood vessels in the legs. This has little effect upon the arterioles, since they have large amounts of smooth muscle and this tissue has the ability to contract in response to a stretching force. By contrast, the veins, which have far less smooth muscle, cannot resist the stretching force from the increased

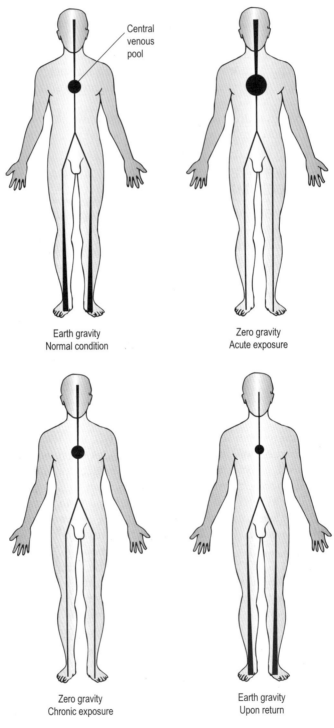

Central
venous
pool

Earth gravity
Normal condition

Zero gravity
Acute exposure

Zero gravity
Chronic exposure

Earth gravity
Upon return

Figure 7.2 Changed 'venous pooling' in different conditions[1]

transmural pressure. They distend and the blood pools in them rather than returning to the heart (Figure 7.2).

The value of G in the above equation need not be due to gravity alone – it refers to the result of any acceleration forces acting upon a column of fluid (the size of the net force being expressed in terms of that due to gravity). In all cases, the pressure increases along the line of acceleration, with the lowest pressure at the 'front'. Thus, if a subject is sitting upright and facing the axis of rotation of a centrifuge, the effect of the acceleration towards the axis of rotation upon the pressures in the blood vessels of the individual make those in his/her back greater than those at his/her front, and these pressures are to be added to those due to the Earth's gravity (pressures in the feet greater than those in the head).

Acceleration forces in addition to those of gravity are generally small and transient – an ascent in a lift, or the 'spring' in a person's gait, for example. Transport has increased these forces, however. In normal journeys by car, the forces due to acceleration, braking and cornering can last for several seconds but are rarely greater than 1-G (that is, an acceleration equal to that exerted by gravity). They act in a backwards or forwards and sideways direction rather than upwards or downwards. Similar forces are experienced in commercial flights. For test pilots and those involved in aerial displays or combat, forces up to 8-G are not uncommon and can act for several seconds. Generally these forces act in a headward direction – as when a plane is turning and the head of the pilot is tilting towards the centre of rotation – but they act in the opposite direction if the pilot is flying 'upside-down' or circling with the head pointing away from the axis of rotation. At fairgrounds, some people seem to enjoy the mixture of fear and exhilaration that accompanies the increased G-forces associated with the rides! Here, the forces are rarely more than 3-G, but they can be experienced for minutes at a time and continually change in the direction in which they are acting.

Decreased G-forces can also be experienced: for example, at the start of a descent in a lift or during a fairground ride, or the drop from the crest of a wave when sailing. Even though patients are subject to normal G-forces, these will act for an extended period of time and in an abnormal direction if they are bedridden. A special case exists when the body is falling freely. In this circumstance, the condition of zero-G or 'weightlessness' is experienced. This phenomenon occurs in the first part of a bungee jump or in freefall parachuting, but will last for a few seconds or minutes only. By contrast, individuals can experience zero-G (or, to be more precise, microgravity) for much longer periods of time if they are in satellites orbiting the Earth, or 'freefalling' in a journey towards the moon or, perhaps in the future, other planets.

From the above, it is clear that changes to the acceleration forces acting on the body, and to the orientation of the body with respect to these forces, will exert effects upon the cardiovascular system as a whole. There will be direct effects upon other physiological systems that are affected by, or respond to, gravity and acceleration forces. These systems include the respiratory and musculo-skeletal systems, and the otoliths and semicircular canals of the vestibular system. Changes in these systems are likely to have repercussions throughout the body, affecting behaviour and renal function, for example.

The question arises how effectively the human body can deal with such changes, both in the short-term and the long-term. Answers to this are relevant to the care of bedridden patients and astronauts; the answers might even determine whether or not humans will be able to travel to other planets and to colonize them.

INCREASED G-FORCES

The advent of rocket travel requires large and continuous acceleration forces to be experienced for several minutes during the launch. Forces of a similar magnitude but in the opposite direction are encountered during re-entry into the Earth's (or any other planet's) atmosphere and landing after a flight. How well human physiology copes with such demands is covered in the next section. The topic has been reviewed by Waterhouse.[2]

Methods of study

If a subject is placed in a large centrifuge, the acceleration force increases in proportion to the speed of rotation and the radius of the turning circle. This acceleration is towards the axis of rotation (centripetal), though the effect of gravity (vertically downwards) is also present. The direction of the overall force acting upon a subject depends upon his/her orientation. Measurements can be made during rotation of the subject, the information being transmitted telemetrically to the experimenters. Most research work has been concerned with the effects of headward acceleration (in which the subject is orientated with the head pointing towards the axis of rotation) upon mental performance and the cardio-respiratory system.

Vision and consciousness

The immediate effects of an acceleration in a headward direction with a force of approximately 4-G causes 'grey-out', a deterioration of both peripheral vision and the perception of colour and detail by the fovea. With a higher acceleration (4.5 to 5-G), vision, but not consciousness, is lost ('black-out'); above 5-G, unconsciousness results.

A detailed explanation of these results does not exist, but it is believed that several factors are involved and contribute to the apparently greater susceptibility of vision. It is likely that chemical factors (the cerebral vasculature shows marked vasomotor responses to changes in the composition of the blood) and anatomical factors (there being some evidence for a decreased distensibility of the veins leaving the skull) are important in the overall responses to acceleration, but this account will concentrate on the pressures in the blood vessels.

The headward acceleration causes a fall in the intraluminal pressure of all

Table 7.1 Summary of the effects of increased G-forces upon vision and consciousness

Force	Effects	Explanation
4-G	'Grey-out' Peripheral vision deteriorates Colour vision is lost	Pressure in retinal vessels falls. This, coupled with intra-ocular pressure, decreases transmural pressure, and the blood vessels begin to reach their 'critical closing pressure' and collapse.
4.5-G	'Black-out' Vision is lost Consciousness maintained	Cerebral vessels are protected in comparison with retinal vessels. Cerebral tissue pressure is determined by cerebrospinal fluid pressure, which, because it too is a column of fluid, changes in parallel to the changes in intravascular pressure. Transmural pressure is maintained, therefore.
>5-G	Consciousness is lost	The intravascular pressure is inadequate to allow the blood to reach the base of the skull.

blood vessels above the heart. In the eye, the retinal arterioles are not protected by the skull and they also pass through the intraocular fluid, which exerts an external pressure on them of about 20 cm H_2O. Both factors reduce the transmural pressure across the retinal arterioles, and their critical closing pressure is reached. The fact that the arterioles radiate outwards from their entry point into the eye, near the macula, means that the vessels supplying the retinal periphery are longer. Increased length is inevitably associated with increased resistance, as a result of which intraluminal pressures in the distal vasculature will tend to be lower and the vessel more likely to fall below its critical closing pressure.

It is suggested that some other aspects of brain function are less susceptible than the eyes to the effects of acceleration (for example, consciousness is maintained during 'black-out') because the cerebral vessels are protected in some way. This protection is believed to arise because the brain is surrounded by an indistensible skull and contains at its centre a column of cerebrospinal fluid. The result of this structural arrangement is that the pressure of the brain tissue surrounding the cerebral vasculature, unlike that of the legs, for example (see above), can differ from that of the atmosphere. Instead, cerebral tissue pressure changes in parallel with changes in the cerebrospinal fluid, another column of fluid. The outcome of this arrangement is that acceleration forces produce similar pressure changes both inside and outside the cerebral blood vessels. That is, for blood vessels in the skull, the transmural pressure and, therefore, vessel size are comparatively unaffected by acceleration forces. The eyes do not benefit from this protection, since their function dictates that they must be outside the skull.

However, when forces in excess of 5-G are experienced, the protective mechanism offered by the skull and cerebrospinal fluid fail, and consciousness is lost. In this circumstance, the blood pressure has largely been dissipated by the time the base of the skull has been reached, and the pressure in the vessels falls below their critical closing pressure. That is, the blood being circulated never reaches the safety provided by the skull and cerebrospinal fluid. Therefore, provided that the vessels below the skull do not collapse, blood flow to the brain is maintained surprisingly well, though deterioration in mental performance before unconsciousness occurs has been measured in some studies. The effects of these changed forces of acceleration are summarized in Table 7.1.

After approximately 5-10 seconds of acceleration, blood flow to the brain and eyes begins to recover, as a result of baroreceptor reflex activity. This reflex activity is also important when acceleration forces are increased only slowly, when it enables cerebral and retinal blood flow to be maintained during forces reaching as high as 6-G. It is likely that the major stimuli are changes in blood pressure monitored by the carotid sinuses, and they induce reflex rises in sympathetic activity and the release of catecholamines into the circulation from the adrenal medulla. The baroreceptors of the aortic arch are likely to be less effective since they are not positioned above the heart. Indeed, it has been suggested that, since these receptors are effectively below the heart, they will monitor a raised blood pressure and so act to reduce the size of the reflex response.

The cardiovascular and respiratory systems

Headward acceleration causes the internal organs of the abdomen to move away from the head; this action pulls the diaphragm in the same direction and so reduces intrathoracic pressure. Even if the force of contraction of the heart and the pulse pressure produced during systole were to remain the same, they would be taking place against this reduction in intrathoracic pressure. As a result, there would be a net fall in the driving force to areas outside the thorax. In practice, the force of contraction of the heart also falls, due to a decreased venous return and the reduced cardiac filling that this causes (according to Starling's law). The fall in venous return is due to an increased pooling of blood in the veins of the dependent parts of the body. This effect is similar to that found on standing up normally (see Figure 7.2), but is more marked because of the increased value of G that is involved. Both of these changes contribute to the fall in blood pressure in the carotid sinus, and this initiates the baroreceptor reflexes.

Acceleration also affects breathing movements and respiratory gas exchange. With headward acceleration, the downward movement of the abdominal organs and the effect of this in displacing the diaphragm downwards facilitate inspiration, but hinder expiration. However, this direction of acceleration also makes it more difficult for the individual to raise the chest wall (part of a normal inspiratory movement) and more easy to lower it (part of the expiratory movement). Since these movements of the rib cage normally contribute less to breathing than do those of the diaphragm,

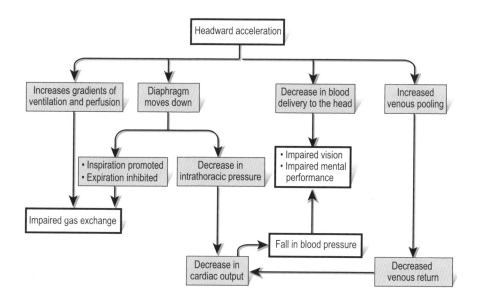

Figure 7.3 Some effects upon the respiratory and cardiovascular systems of headward acceleration

the net effect upon breathing is to make inspiration easier and to emphasize the role of movements of the diaphragm. Tidal volume tends to encroach upon the inspiratory reserve. Acceleration away from the head produces the opposite effects, inspiration now becoming more difficult.

The lungs normally show gradients of blood perfusion and alveolar ventilation; in a normal 1-G environment, both increase from the apex to the base. These gradients are both produced by factors which are affected by acceleration forces. Therefore, acceleration in a headward direction accentuates the gradients whereas acceleration in the opposite direction can reverse them. During headward acceleration, the apical alveoli will be almost fully distended throughout the respiratory cycle but receive very little ventilation and even zero perfusion; therefore, their ventilation/perfusion ratio will be abnormally high. By contrast, the pulmonary vessels at the base of the lung have increased pressures (so much so that there is even the possibility of pulmonary oedema) and receive large amounts of blood. Even though ventilation rises, it does not do so proportionally and a lowered ventilation/perfusion ratio at the base of the lungs is the outcome. As a result of these gradients in the ventilation/perfusion ratio, the apex and base of the lung function poorly with respect to gas exchange. Alveolar deadspace at the apex and venous shunts at the base cause ventilatory effort and cardiac work, respectively, to be wasted, and hypoxaemia and even ischaemia develop.

Some of the effects of headward acceleration upon the cardiovascular and respiratory systems are shown in Figure 7.3.

Countermeasures

Many of the cardiovascular problems associated with acceleration are caused by the redistribution of blood flow. This redistribution arises because intraluminal pressures change in accord with the term h.p.G in the equation above (where h represents the distance between the heart and the site under consideration as measured along the direction of acceleration), whereas pressures outside the vessels (except in the case of the cerebrospinal fluid and brain tissue, see Table 7.1) do not change. This knowledge enables countermeasures to be considered – measures that decrease h or change extravascular tissue pressure by a similar amount.

If it is possible for a person to accelerate 'forwards' rather than headwards, pressure gradients will be lessened because the thickness of the body is less than its height, and so h is decreased. This requirement means the astronaut or pilot ought to be in a supine rather than a sitting position. There are obvious implications for the design of the cockpit or space capsule, and some degree of compromise might be called for if vision outside is required. When the orientation of the body is changed in this way, a greater tolerance to G-forces has been found, and the fall in venous return is reduced. These changes in orientation will also decrease the difficulties associated with breathing and the excessive ventilation/perfusion imbalances.

Other means exist to oppose the fall in cardiac output. It can be prevented transiently by performing a Valsalva manoeuvre (that is, a forced expiration against a closed epiglottis), by shouting, or by positive-pressure breathing. All these methods are effective for a few heartbeats because they raise intra-thoracic pressure and so maintain the 'baseline' pressure upon which the heart operates. Often, this might be sufficient.

If the countermeasure is needed to act for more than a few seconds, and this will be the case for astronauts, then further measures become necessary to maintain venous return. These can include tensing the leg and thigh muscles, though this is not possible when the legs are required for other purposes, such as piloting a helicopter. In principle, and analogous to the conditions that exist in the skull (see Table 7.1), if changes in tissue pressure in the legs and abdomen could match changes in intraluminal pressure, then the transmural pressure across blood vessels could be maintained at normal values, and this would prevent pooling of blood in the veins.

Theoretically, encasing the lower body in an indistensible covering would achieve this, since any distension of the blood vessels would cause the lower body to expand, and the indistensible casing would result in an equal rise of tissue pressure, so preventing the increase in the transmural pressure. This 'solution' would be quite impracticable, of course, due to the immobility and discomfort that it would produce. An alternative method would be to surround the lower body with a water bath, changes in intraluminal pressure being reflected in the changes in water pressure and tissue pressure. (This is, in effect, the position with regard to the relationship between cerebral blood vessels, brain tissue and the cerebrospinal fluid.) This method is unacceptable also, if only because of the need to minimize the payload of a rocket as much

Box 7.1 Some countermeasures to the effects of increased acceleration forces

Short-term measures:
Singing, shouting, and performing the Valsalva manoeuvre: these maintain intrathoracic pressure - but reduce venous return.
Tensing and contracting the leg muscles: this reduces the fall in venous return (the 'muscle pump') - but precludes the performance of tasks which require coordinated leg movement.

Longer-term measures:
Changed orientation: this reduces the value of 'h' in the term h.p.G - but it can compromise the type of task that can be performed.
Antigravity suit: this prevents tissue distension and so raises tissue pressure and prevents the rise in transmural pressure - but it can be too cumbersome for continuous use.

as possible. However, the 'antigravity suit' has been designed to achieve the same effects as the water bath. It does not encase the lower body completely, and is air-filled rather than filled with water, but it acts by raising the pressure outside the lower body, which, in turn, raises tissue pressure. It is an effective countermeasure, not only because the suit prevents venous pooling but also because it limits the descent of the diaphragm. This decrease in the amount by which the diaphragm descends maintains the heart nearer to the head, so decreasing the value of h and the amount of pressure required to drive blood up to the brain. The combination of a changed orientation of the subject, of muscle contraction, and the use of an antigravity suit has been shown to be most effective.

A further countermeasure can be taken to reduce visual disturbances. Goggles can be worn that enable the extra-ocular pressure (and, hence, the pressure surrounding the retinal vessels) to be changed. Decreases in extra-ocular pressure act to promote retinal blood flow and combat high G-forces in the headward direction, by maintaining the transmural pressure gradient in the retinal vessels. In effect, the goggles are acting as a miniature antigravity suit for the eyes but, since the eyes are above the head, they change pressures in the opposite direction. Conversely, if the pilot is flying upside-down, so that retinal intravascular pressure and the transmural pressure gradient are increased, raised pressure in the goggles maintains the transmural pressure gradient at normal values – directly analogous to the effects of an antigravity suit worn around the lower body in subjects accelerating upwards.

These countermeasures are summarised in Box 7.1.

PHYSIOLOGICAL EFFECTS OF WEIGHTLESSNESS

If humans are to explore the solar system, they will have to endure weightlessness for years. For example, with current technology, the trip to Mars and back would take about two years. What changes take place when humans live in a zero-G (microgravity) environment for extended periods? Can they be said to adjust to such periods of zero-G? If so, what happens when they return to live again in a gravitational field, whether back on Earth or on another planet? Such questions apply at the moment to a very restricted number of people, but a similar problem exists for the much greater number of patients who are bedridden for extended periods of time. Even though they are still subject to gravity, it no longer acts along the length of their bodies. What changes occur in these patients, and what happens when they have recovered enough to stand and walk again?

Means of study

The force of gravity on Earth is ubiquitous and its effects are difficult to remove for extended periods of time. The effects can be removed transiently if a subject is in 'freefall'. Parabolic flights can achieve this state under controlled conditions. Subjects are put in a plane that flies in a parabolic curve towards the ground. This enables zero-G to be experienced for about 30 seconds before the pilot has to pull the plane up out of the dive. However, before the first manned space flights, it was necessary to have some idea of how astronauts would react to weightlessness over a period of at least a few days.

Investigations on Earth use constant bed rest and water-immersion techniques to mimic the effects of weightlessness. When using a complete bed rest regimen, it is better to have the volunteers tilted at $6°$ to the horizontal with their head down (head-down tilt) rather than in a horizontal posture. This is for anatomical reasons; in this position, the carotid sinuses become level with the aortic valve, rather than slightly above it. This reduces h to zero, so that the pressure difference (h.p.G) is zero and so mimics the effects of zero-G more accurately. Studies lasting up to about a year have been performed using this method. A major difficulty with it is in deciding what changes in posture should be allowed for meals and toilet and for carrying out tasks that might be required in space.

Patients who have been immobilized during recovery from ligament operations also provide useful information, but patients recovering from bone fractures or coma are less useful because of the interpretive difficulties that might arise. A comatose patient can hardly be regarded as 'normal' and there would be considerable doubts as to how 'normal' were any bone changes (see below) in somebody recovering from a fracture.

The rationale for water-immersion studies is that, since the individual floats, the force of gravity is completely opposed by the upthrust exerted by the water – the subject is, in effect, 'weightless'. This method suffers from several problems. The temperature of the water affects considerably the subject's comfort; heat transfer between the body and water is more rapid than that between the body and dry air (water is far less of a thermal insulator than air), and the evaporation of sweat is not possible. Also, the subject needs to be separated from the water by an impervious sheet, to prevent damage to the skin and tissue oedema due to water uptake; besides, movement under water is difficult because of its viscosity. Nevertheless, water immersion provides an environment in which the difficulties of exerting a force upon an object – difficulties that arise because of the problem of getting the purchase required to be able to exert such a force – can be experienced.

Animal models, involving total body suspension, tail suspension and hindlimb suspension, have also been used.[3] In the first model, the load is removed from all four limbs; in the others, from the hind limbs only, and the animal is free to move around the cage. The hindlimb suspension model has the advantage that the forelimbs can be used as controls for changes to the hindlimbs. However, since the animals used, mainly rats, are quadrupeds, the results might not translate easily from them when changed vestibular reflexes and the effects of spinal unloading are considered in bipedal humans.

In spite of these problems, results from the above types of study are similar to those obtained so far, from animals and humans, in the prolonged space flights (up to one year) of the Soyuz, Salyut, Skylab, Mir and Spacelab programmes. For this reason, the results from all techniques can be assumed to be similar unless it is stated otherwise. Moreover, the recent increase in co-operative ventures between nations, and the much more widespread dissemination of results to the scientific community as a whole, have both meant that the body of common knowledge has increased enormously in recent years.

One method of investigating the response to living in space consists of measuring changes that occur in the astronauts while still in the zero-G environment; but this is difficult due to lack of space and time, and the highly technical apparatus that can be required. The more common alternative is to assess astronauts as soon as possible after their return to Earth. In this case, however, it must be remembered that individuals have been exposed to the deceleration forces associated with re-entry into the Earth's atmosphere and landing, and that it is not always possible to conduct tests immediately after landing. That is, if re-adjustments to the effects of deceleration forces and gravity are rapid, the observed results will reflect this response as well as the original effects of weightlessness.

Body fluids

During weightlessness in space and head-down body tilt, there is a redistribution of approximately 2 l of body fluids away from the dependent parts of the body and towards the head, neck and thorax.[4,5] This loss of venous pooling is caused by the decrease of the transmural pressure gradient across the veins, the value of h.p.G being at, or very close to, zero. For approximately the first three days in space, astronauts report that the head and neck feel bloated, often with an increased incidence of headaches, the neck veins become engorged and the legs become thinner – the 'chicken-leg syndrome'. These immediate changes are illustrated in Figure 7.2. After some days in space, the total loss of body fluids is up to about 6 l; little of this comes from the chest region, about 0.5 l from the lower torso, 1.5-2.0 l from the thighs, and 1.5 l from the calves (the source of the other fluid is unclear).

During this period, it would be predicted from a consideration of the increased return of blood to the volume receptors in the atria and great veins that there would be an increase in the central venous pool and central venous pressure, leading to a marked diuresis (the Gauer-Henry reflex). Further, it would be predicted that there would be a decrease in antidiuretic hormone secretion, decreased activity of the renin-angiotensin-aldosterone axis, and an increase in atrial natriuretic peptide secretion, all of which would promote fluid loss from the body. In practice, many of these changes have been difficult to demonstrate.[6] A diuresis has been measured in some, but by no means all, flights. A more common finding has been a decline in urine flow to lower levels than normal. Moreover, the predicted changes in the patterns of hormone secretion have not been demonstrated unambiguously. Finally, even though there is an increase in the central venous pool, it is not invariably associated with an increase in central venous filling pressure. In short, even though the role of the Gauer-Henry reflex is well established on Earth-bound studies, other factors seem to be imporatant in the zero-G environment.

The fall in urine production is probably due, at least in part, to the decreased fluid intake that is common before and during flights. Whether this fall in fluid intake results from a fall in the sensation of thirst, or indicates instead an intentional decrease in fluid intake to reduce the inconvenience of emptying the bladder in a zero-G environment – or reflects some other mechanism – is not entirely clear.

In water-immersion studies lasting several days, there is, by contrast, a marked diuresis. This is attributed to compression of the tissues in conjunction with a loss of pooling of blood in the veins of the dependent parts of the body. This result raises the question of the possible role that tissue pressure and the distensibility of tissue play in any redistribution of body fluids and reflex changes in urine production that occur in these circumstances. In a zero-G environment, tissue pressure in the dependent parts of the body is likely to fall, particularly if muscle tone decreases also (which is likely to be the case as there is now no need to support the body's weight). This drop would reduce the return of blood to the heart, and so damp down those reflexes that lead to the loss of body fluids. Even so, the distensibility of the tissue of the chest wall, neck and face is higher than that of the legs and thighs, and this would be predicted to contribute to the initial thinning of the legs and thighs, and engorgement of the tissues in the upper parts of the body. It is not clear if these differences in distensibility become less with time spent in zero-G.

Whatever the detailed mechanisms involved, the changes in fluid distribution result in a correction of the excess in the thoracic veins, and so reduce the pre-load on the heart due to increased filling. The position reached after the correction has taken place is summarized by Figure 7.2.

The cardiovascular system

Initially, weightlessness causes an increase in cardiac output due to the lack of venous pooling and increased return of blood to the heart.[5,7] Blood pressure

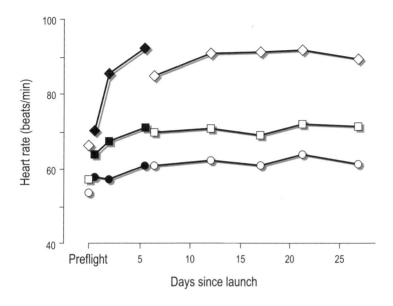

Figure 7.4 The mean heart rate, before and during flight, measured at rest (circles) and in response to lower body negative pressure of 30 mmHg (squares) or 50 mmHg (diamonds). Results from Skylab missions shown as open figures, from Shuttle flights as closed ones.[8]

rises, but there is likely to be a contribution from the stress associated with space flight. After correction of the increase in venous return (see above), blood pressure, cardiac output and heart rate fall towards normal values, though heart rate continues to be elevated. This rise might reflect the fact that blood volume is slightly decreased, and so venous return, cardiac output and blood pressure can be maintained only by increasing sympathetic outflow. This increased neural activity might also decrease the distensibility of the veins in the legs, so off-setting the effects of the fall in tissue pressure described above.

Some reports suggest that, with longer periods of weightlessness (over 50 days), the heart becomes smaller. This decrease has been attributed to atrophy of the cardiac muscle, though other reports suggest that this is not the case but rather the chambers of the heart become smaller due to decreased filling.

There is some evidence for cardiovascular 'deconditioning' under prolonged zero-G conditions, as can be seen when the responses to circulatory 'stresses' are considered (see Figure 7.4). Thus, the cardiovascular changes produced by exercise after time spent in space are more marked than observed before the flight. Also, after experimentally decreasing venous return (for example, by inflating cuffs around the thighs), the time that elapses before fainting occurs is decreased. Many of the changes are believed to be caused by changes to the sensitivity of the baroreceptor reflexes and to the balance between sympathetic and parasympathetic tone.

The respiratory system

When standing upright on Earth, there are gradients of perfusion and ventilation from the apex down to the base of the lungs. Both gradients are due in part to the effects of gravity, and they result in an uneven ventilation-perfusion ratio and a decreased efficiency of the lungs with regard to gas exchange (see Figure 7.3). In a zero-G environment, these imbalances become much smaller, as would be predicted, but they do not disappear.[9,10] This is believed to be due to local differences in the distensibility of the lung tissue.

The distribution of particles inhaled into the lungs depends upon their size and, with the larger particles, is affected by gravity. There are many air-borne particles in the space cabin environment – both from the cabin itself and from its occupants – and many of these particles will carry microbes. In the absence of gravity, such particles are likely to pass further into the lungs. Whether this increases the chances of infection is not yet known.

It is the current practice for astronauts performing extra-vehicular activities to wear a suit which contains only oxygen to breathe. In this way, the pressure of gas in the suit can be low, so increasing the suit's manoeuvrability. However, the cabin atmosphere also contains nitrogen, and so there is the risk that bubbles of nitrogen will appear in the astronauts' blood when they change to pure oxygen from the cabin mixture – this is similar to the problem that deep-sea divers face on resurfacing, and is called the 'bends'. In both environments the decompression problems are overcome by 'decompression routines'. Such routines are time-consuming, however, and the development of suits which remain flexible when filled with the same gas mixture used in the cabin is a priority.

The vestibular system

Many astronauts experience giddiness, spatial disorientation, nausea, and even vomiting during the first few days in space. Some, especially if they move their head, have symptoms of kinaesthesia – illusions of moving or falling – and there is a transient deterioration of hand-eye coordination.[11-14] These symptoms are attributed to a change in the balance between the different neural inputs that normally reach the brain in the presence of 1-G forces (Figure 7.5). The input from the semicircular canals (which indicates angular acceleration) is similar to that found on Earth, the inputs from the muscle, tendon and joint receptors (which signal the postural forces acting on the body) will be modified in the weightless condition, and the otolith receptors (which signal the orientation of the head in the gravitational field) will become far less active (Figure 7.5). Similar problems, also attributed to an abnormal mixture of inputs to the brain, can be produced on Earth by spending time in a rough sea on board ship (sea-sickness) and by prolonged rides at the fairground ('All the fun of the fair').

Attempts to predict, from the results of experiments performed on Earth and investigating vestibulo-ocular and opto-kinetic reflexes, those astronauts in whom problems in space will be most severe have so far met with only

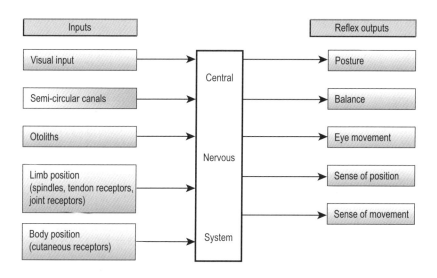

Figure 7.5 Inputs controlling posture, balance and associated sensations

limited success. One possible test is to compare the reflex movements of the eyes which oppose the effects of a change in head position; if the sizes of the responses to moving the head to the right or left are unequal, then there is evidence that the individual might be more prone to space sickness.

Nausea is not observed during water-immersion and bed rest studies. This is because the abnormal balance of inputs does not occur in such circumstances, the force of gravity still being present. This shows again the problems associated with an extrapolation of results obtained from studies simulating the condition of weightlessness to the real experience of space flight.

On Earth, information from the otoliths in the inner ear, from the joints, tendons and stretch receptors in the muscles, and from the visual input are all integrated to give information about 'up' and 'down'. In zero-G, much of this information is absent, and expressions such as 'stand upright, with your feet down on the floor' and 'lie down and go to sleep' become almost meaningless. 'Up' and 'down' have to be redefined in the space cabin environment, and more use has to be made of visual clues. All of this requires mental adjustment by the astronaut and, until this is achieved, will contribute to the initial disorientation.

Even after any such adjustment has been made, the altered balance between the inputs from the different receptors remains. Much of the evidence attests to the plasticity of the brain, with opto-kinetic reflexes becoming more important than vestibulo-spinal ones. That is, the central nervous system becomes influenced more by visual inputs than when on Earth, and 'learns' to re-interpret the changed inputs from the sense organs so that the astronaut can continue to perform co-ordinated movements. There is also a limited amount of evidence, generally from animals, indicating that there are changes in the activity of afferent pathways from the vestibular apparatus. These findings suggest that an increased input from the semicircular canals, rather than the otoliths, develops in space. Whether this change reflects changes to the receptors themselves and/or to their efferent control is unclear; in either case, it can be seen as an example of the CNS placing an increased emphasis upon those receptors that provide useful information in the space environment (Figure 7.5).

All objects, not just astronauts, are weightless in zero-G and yet their inertial properties, due to mass, are unchanged. For example, to hold a large hammer in a zero-G environment requires no effort, but to swing it to strike an object requires the same force as on Earth. This is initially disconcerting for the astronaut. The astronaut therefore learns to make much more use of inertial clues. Such clues are, in fact, used on Earth when estimating the weight of objects, as when the object is placed on the hand and the hand is moved up and down. (This method is effective because the weight of an object in a gravitational field is directly related to its mass.) There is the added difficulty in a zero-G environment that the act of swinging the hammer will cause the astronaut to rotate in the opposite direction – 'to every action, there is an equal and opposite reaction' – unless he/she is strapped to some immovable object.

The musculo-skeletal system

Movement is limited by lack of space available to the astronauts, and there is also far less need for tonic activity in the 'antigravity' extensor muscles – on Earth, those in the spine are active for about 16 hours per day. It is not surprising, therefore, that some muscular atrophy occurs, as indicated by direct measures of strength and fatigue, and by the increased excretion of urea in the urine.[15,16] The atrophy seems to be due to a reduction in the cross-sectional area of fibres rather than their number. Even so, not all muscles and muscle types are affected equally. The muscles affected most are, as might be predicted, the slow extensor muscles, those that normally bear the weight of the body. By contrast, fast flexor muscles are least affected, and fast extensor muscles are affected by an intermediate amount. When the proportions of different types of fibre in a muscle are examined, slow, fatigue-resistant fibres decrease and fast, fatiguing fibres increase. Metabolically, there is a shift from fibres that derive energy from oxidative phosphorylation to those that derive it glycolytically.

Muscle and tendon reflexes change also. There is evidence, often from animal studies, that muscle spindles become more sensitive to changing length, that there are changes in the motor neurone pool affected reflexly by these organs, and that the threshold for the Achilles tendon reflex decreases.

Bones begin to demineralize during a stay in zero-G.[17-22] This loss of bone material can be measured directly from densitometry studies of individual bones, or indirectly from the rates of urinary excretion of hydroxyproline and calcium. As with muscles, not all bones are affected equally; the loss of mineral is greatest from those bones that normally bear the weight of the body but, even in these, the regions near to the tendon insertions tend to be affected less. If Earth-bound studies use prolonged immobility as a model (encasing the bones in plaster, for example), it is observed that there is no difference between the responses of those bones that normally bear weight and those that do not. This model has therefore proved to be of very limited value for such investigations.

Interest has focused also on the process of bone remodelling, which results from the integration of formation and reabsorption processes by osteoblasts and osteoclasts, respectively. Changes in the activity of both of these cell types have been reported, together with a loss of the normal coupling that exists between them. Since the process of remodelling is related in some way to the physical stresses experienced by bone, these findings are not unexpected. Nevertheless, the calcification of cartilage does not appear to be affected, chick embryos appearing to show normal osteogenesis.

Studies of changes to those hormones associated with bone metabolism – parathyroid hormone and 1,25-dihydroxy vitamin D (which mobilize calcium from bone) and calcitonin (which inhibits bone resorption by osteoclasts) – have produced inconsistent results, and the picture is very unclear.[6,17,23]

The position is complicated by the possibilities that the sensitivity of tissues to these hormones might alter and that local hormones might be involved instead or in addition to the blood-borne ones. However, a more consistent view is that the decreased uptake of calcium from the gut contributes to the process of demineralization.

An alarming finding is that the rate at which minerals are lost from those bones that are affected is approximately 0.5 per cent of the total per month, and that the process is not checked. It appears to continue at an unchanging rate during 6 months of bed rest or during space flights of approximately one year (the longest times so far studied). If the process turns out not to be self-limiting, this result implies a considerable danger of bone fractures on return to a normal, 1-G environment after approximately two years in space – barely sufficient time for a round trip to Mars, for example.

One other effect of bone resorption is the increased loss of calcium in the urine. Coupled with the low rates of drinking and urine production in astronauts (see above), there is an increase in calcium concentration in the urine. This increase explains the greater production of renal calculi (insoluble 'stones' containing calcium salts) that has been observed, and implies that there is an increased medical risk to the astronaut.

Other systems and factors

The red and white blood cell counts fall in zero-G. Since cell breakdown does not seem to change, this implies that production falls by more than the decrease in plasma volume. Indeed, for an unknown reason, bone marrow activity almost ceases, at least during the first days of weightlessness. In addition, the immune response is damped[24,25] and there is a re-activation of some dormant viruses. The effects of such depressed immune responses upon the longer-term health of astronauts have still to be assessed.

Box 7.2 Changes during zero-G

A. Areas where changes can be regarded as beneficial and part of acclimatization
Body fluids - loss of excess fluid due to lack of pooling of blood
Cardiovascular system - decreased blood volume and heart activity due to lack of postural effects
Respiratory system - improved ventilation/perfusion balance
Skeletal muscle - loss of muscle that is excess to reduced postural requirements
Bone - loss of calcium that is excess due to reduced postural stresses
Balance and postural reflexes - increased emphasis upon inputs from vision and angular acceleration

B. Areas where there might be problems (but more data are required)
Immune responses - these are reduced; are there long-term problems?
Haemopoiesis - erythrocyte production falls
Ionizing radiation - long-term exposure levels that are safe are unknown
Psychology - the long-term effects of isolation are unknown
Medicine - greater problems exist for minor operations, and full treatment of major disorders is impossible
Reproduction - is this possible, and is embryogenesis unaltered?

Whilst not within the remit of an account of the physiological responses to weightlessness, it deserves mention that there will be considerable psychological burdens upon astronauts venturing out into the solar system. The effects of radiation will also need to be considered; protection against this (e.g. use of lead) is difficult and expensive to incorporate into the design of spacecraft. A balance has to be struck between the minimum protection that can still be regarded as 'safe' and the cost of providing this protection.

Any medical help will have to be provided on board the spacecraft. Minor operations in zero-G conditions can be more complex than on Earth, if only because blood lost by bleeding no longer collects on the surface of the patient. More complex operations will pose greater difficulties and stresses. During the course of a mission lasting several years and with a crew of 10 persons, for example, such an emergency becomes, from a statistical viewpoint, much more than only a remote possibility. Difficult decisions about what to do in such circumstances, and even, possibly, how to deal with a deceased crew member, will have to be made.

Acclimatization to zero–G

Zero gravity provides a very different environment from that on Earth, and the above account outlines the changes that have been observed in astronauts and in experiments on Earth upon volunteers and animals. Many of the changes can be seen as a process of acclimatization to this new environment, one in which many aspects of workload are reduced.

For example, the amount of work that needs to be performed by the heart is decreased, there no longer being alterations of pressure caused by postural changes. In such circumstances, any changes to the heart that might take place are being misinterpreted if they are described as 'deconditioning'. Similarly, removal of excess body fluids, decreases in extensor muscle strength, changes in muscle metabolism, changes in the vestibular system and its reflexes, and the loss of calcium from bone (calcium is a valuable resource, and the amount of it in our Earth-bound bones is far in excess of what is needed in space) – all of these result in a human body more attuned to zero-G than the one that left Earth.

It can be argued, therefore, that humans can adjust to zero-G, but there are other areas where the changes observed do not seem to be advantageous; the decreased activity of the immune system is one example. There are also many areas (the individual's psychology, the ability to reproduce, and the human's susceptibility to ionizing radiation, for example), where far more data are required. From our current perspective, however, it does not seem that the physiology of humans is such that space travel is impossible (see Box 7.2).

The return to Earth

Such optimism must be tempered by the knowledge that the individual must then return to Earth, or land on some other planet. This return will re-expose the astronaut to gravitational forces once again. The size of these depends upon the size and composition of the planet, of course, and the difficulties will be proportional to the size of the new gravitational field. What is required is a knowledge of how disadvantaged the astronaut will now be, together with an understanding of how rapidly acclimatization to the new gravitational forces can be achieved.

The potential hazard from bone demineralization[17] has been mentioned already, but other problems exist. On return to an upright posture, blood once again pools in the dependent parts of the body (see Figure 7.2). Bearing in mind that the blood volume is decreased by at least 10 per cent, that tissue distensibility might be changed, and that the cardiovascular system might show signs of 'deconditioning', the potential difficulties of standing upright and exercising become obvious. Decreased tolerance of the cardiovascular system to the stresses imposed by standing upright (orthostatic hypotension) and by taking exercise immediately after the return to Earth, have been observed (Figure 7.4). Astronauts show pre-syncope symptoms, and some actually faint in the days immediately after return to Earth.[5] Gradients of ventilation and perfusion reappear in the lungs, their efficiency thereby decreasing.[9] Weakened skeletal muscles, particularly the tonic extensors, become fatigued as they are required, once again, to support the weight of the body.[15] Postural reflexes are exaggerated and the posture and gait are abnormal,[11] due to the 'resetting' of the vestibular and opto-kinetic reflexes that has taken place (Figure 7.5).

In short, the returned astronaut is an enfeebled creature, needing help to stand and to walk, and suffering from disorientation and postural instability,

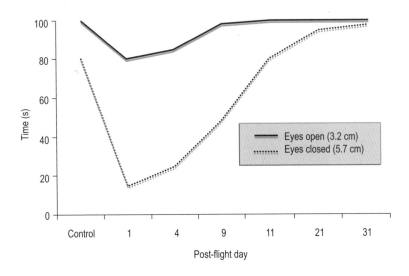

Figure 7.6 Mean time-courses of recovery of balance after space flights lasting 59–84 days. Astronauts were tested before the flight (Control) and on several occasions after their return to Earth. The test consisted of measuring how long (up to a maximum of 100 s) individuals could maintain their balance on a narrow (3.2 cm) or wide (5.7 cm) beam with their eyes open or closed.[26]

particularly in the dark or if the eyes are closed (see below). The cardiovascular, muscular and skeletal problems, but not those associated with balance (since they have remained in a gravitational field), are found also in previously bedridden patients starting to stand and walk again.

The individual immediately begins the process of acclimatization to the new environment. In the days following their return, astronauts drink copiously, their kidneys conserve salt, and the number of circulating reticulocytes increases as the anaemia due to the previous, low haemopoietic activity of the bone marrow is corrected. The functions of the vestibular and opto-kinetic reflexes begin to be re-established, and the individual regains a conventional posture and gait. Some of these changes are rapid, but the ability to maintain one's balance in the absence of visual information takes longer, up to 10 days (Figure 7.6). The rate of recovery of skeletal muscle has not been studied at all fully but it is essentially complete after 5 months, and astronauts have undertaken subsequent flights without evidence of residual ill-effects from an earlier flight.

The position is less clear, however, with regard to the recalcification of bone. The time-course of the correction of osteoporosis is unclear, and the relative importance in this recovery of bone formation and resorption, of calcitonin, 1,25-dihydroxy vitamin D, and parathyroid hormone, are all areas where adequate data have yet to be obtained.[17]

Counter-measures to zero-G and other preparations for the return to Earth

Clearly, acclimatization to a zero-G environment is ill-advised if the traveller wishes to return to Earth, or to visit some other planet. Much effort has gone into minimizing the unpleasant side-effects found in the first days after exposure to zero-G. As an example of such a countermeasure, since nausea immediately after arrival in space is most marked following a head movement, some Russian astronauts have worn caps that restrict such movement. In the longer term, methods have aimed at opposing some of the changes associated with acclimation to zero-G (see Box 7.3). These methods have aimed particularly at preventing changes to the cardiovascular and musculo-skeletal systems. They can be divided into those that attempt to mimic the effects of gravity and those that attempt to replace some of the effects of gravity by instituting programmes of exercise.[4,27,28]

Lower body negative pressure (LBNP) is a method by which a suction device is applied around the legs and thighs. This procedure causes blood to pool in the legs and so decreases venous return, thereby mimicking the normal orthostatic stress that occurs when standing upright in a 1-G environment. Investigators have tried to establish how great a negative pressure is required, and for how long. A 4-hour period with a LBNP of -30 mmHg has been used, for example, but there is some evidence that 4 x 1 hour per day of such treatment is more effective than 1 x 4 hour per day. The apparatus is cumbersome, however, and it also is an inexact mimic of the position that exists on Earth. The pressure inside the apparatus is uniformly low whereas, on Earth, there is a gradient of pressure along the length of the leg due to pressure gradients within the columns of blood.

Exercise is used to combat changes to the skeleton and its musculature, and possible changes to the heart. It must be emphasized that conventional training methods and apparatus are often worthless in a zero-G environment, where there is no reaction between a weightless subject and a treadmill, and 'weights' are weightless (though it still requires a force to move them and overcome their inertia). Therefore, exercise apparatus in these conditions either requires the subject to be strapped into the device or it has to be designed so that one muscle group can pull against another. Methods used include the cycle ergometer, springs, or isometric contractions. Questions about how much exercise is needed and the most effective type of exercise are currently being investigated. Again, it appears that several short bouts of exercise are more effective than a single longer one.

It has also been suggested that the diet of astronauts needs to be re-evaluated, with the possibility of calcium and vitamin D supplementation.[29-31] This regimen is successful in combating osteoporosis in post-menopausal women, for example. Also, exercise combined with administration of ethane-1-hydroxy-1-diphosphonate (an inhibitor of bone resorption) has been found to reduce the loss of bone calcium.

One of the basic problems is that planetary gravity exerts its effects continuously, and that the effects of sitting or standing will be exerted for

Box 7.3 Some countermeasures to the effects of zero-G

Lower Body Negative Pressure (LBNP) - this is designed to mimic the effects of gravity by causing pooling of the blood in the lower limbs. Four sessions per day, of 1 h each with a pressure of -30 mmHg, is commonly used.

Exercise - the astronaut must be tied down to any treadmill by elastic bands, or perform isometric contractions or contractions against frictional loads. Again, several short bouts of exercise are preferred to a single long one.

Diet - supplementation of the diet with calcium and Vitamin D, in an attempt to reduce demineralisation of bone, is recommended.

Wearing Special Garments - these are designed with springs that need to be opposed continuously by muscle effort, or of a material that requires extra effort to be made whenever a movement is performed. Both reduce the abilities to perform fine and coordinated movements.

Centrifugal Force - this has not been investigated yet but, with larger space stations, the speed of rotation required to produce a given centrifugal force will not need to be as great as is the case with stations currently in use. However, the size of the force and the proportion of the 24 h that it needs to be in operation have not been determined.

about 16 hours per day. To duplicate these effects of gravity in space would require the creation of an artificial gravity by imparting a spin (and, hence, centrifugal force) to the spacecraft. The size of centrifugal force needed to prevent the observed changes is not known. Since centrifugal force is proportional to the radius of rotation as well as the angular velocity, if the force required is at all substantial, then the angular velocity of a small spacecraft (but not a large space station) might be unacceptably large to allow for navigation and routine manoeuvres.

Attempts to provide appropriate stresses for the musculo-skeletal system throughout the waking period have been made by requiring the astronauts to wear 'constant-load suits' – also known as 'Penguin suits' and 'Chibis suits'. These require the continuous expenditure of muscular effort – to oppose springs that are incorporated into the arms and legs of the suit, or increased effort to make a movement, due to the stiffness of the material from which the suit is made. Such garments will compromise co-ordinated movements in general, of course, and fine movements might no longer be possible.

All these methods (with the exception of artificial gravity, which has not yet been investigated) have some value in reducing the 'deconditioning' that extended life in space produces. Post-flight investigations indicate that these measures reduce the cardiovascular changes, and decrease many of the difficulties due to postural orthostasis after returning to Earth. However, the changes in erythropoiesis and vestibular function, and the atrophy of skeletal muscle and bone, are by no means completely prevented. The current view is that a combination of methods is best, if only because it is less boring for the astronauts (Box 7.3). Certainly, as the experience of living in space has increased, there has been a tendency to use several methods regularly, these reducing many of the undesirable effects. However, the problem of bone resorption continues to be the most intractable.

It is clear that much further work is needed to establish the most appropriate combination of countermeasures for astronauts whose stay in a zero-G environment is a prolonged one.

For bedridden patients, many of the above countermeasures are often inappropriate, and so the process of deconditioning can go unchecked. However, attempts to try a limited range of exercises while still in bed seem worth investigation. Even if such exercises are carried out, it is necessary for the patients to be strictly supervised and to undergo appropriate physiotherapy during their first days after getting up.

Just before astronauts return to Earth, extra measures are taken to prepare them for the increased forces associated with the deceleration produced by re-entry into the Earth's atmosphere. Astronauts wear 'antigravity suits' once again (to minimize the pooling of body fluids that will take place (Figure 7.2) and their body fluid volume is deliberately expanded by requiring them to drink saline.[8]

OVERVIEW

Astronauts face many physiological challenges during the course of launch, a sojourn in space and the return to Earth. Many of the problems arise because of the large acceleration and deceleration forces experienced during the launch and landing, and because of exposure to the microgravity environment during much of the flight. A knowledge of hydrostatics has proved invaluable to an understanding of some of the problems encountered.

During the launch, the problem is one of maintaining a blood supply to the brain, eyes and muscles that is sufficient to allow purposeful activities to be continued, or even to prevent the death of the astronaut. In practice, appropriate orientation of the astronaut with respect to the direction of acceleration, coupled with the wearing of protective space suits, enables this to be achieved.

During the extended period of microgravity, changes take place in the neuromuscular, cardio-respiratory and musculo-skeletal systems, many of which can be regarded as appropriate adjustments to the reduced demands placed upon these systems by the microgravity environment. The reduced demands would include lower work-loads for the postural muscles and heart, and reduced stresses on those parts of the skeleton that support a bipedal posture. The evidence suggests that humans can adjust to such an environment.

The problems arise on landing back on Earth, when the changes that took place during exposure to microgravity are inappropriate to living in a 1-G gravitational field. Whilst some of the difficulties can be ameliorated by requiring the astronaut to perform exercise and wear special clothing when in space, there is still concern about the ability to deal effectively with the demineralization of some bones that appears to continue throughout the time spent in microgravity. The outstanding problems need to be solved if humans are to leave the Earth for extended periods of time, as is required by interplanetary travel, and they currently provide an area of active research.

References

1. Howard P. Acceleration. In: The principles and practice of human physiology. Edholm OG, Weiner JS (eds). London: Academic Press, 1982
2. Waterhouse JM. Acceleration forces. In: Human physiology: age, stress and the environment. Case RM, Waterhouse JM (eds). Oxford: Oxford Science Publications, 1993
3. Tipton CM. Animal models and their importance to human physiological responses in microgravity. Med Sci Sports Exerc 1996; 28:S94-S100
4. Baisch FJ. Body fluid distribution in man in space and effect of lower body negative pressure treatment. Clin Inv 1993; 71:690-699
5. Watenpugh DE, Hargens AR. The cardiovascular system in microgravity In: Handbook of physiology. Section 4: Environmental physiology. Volume I. Fregly MJ, Blatteis CM (eds). Oxford: Oxford University Press, 1996:631-674
6. Strollo F. Hormonal changes in humans during spaceflight. Adv Space Biol Med 1999; 7: 99-129
7. Charles JB, Lathers CM. Cardiovascular adaptation to space flight. J Clin Pharmacol 1991; 31:1010-1023
8. Charles JB, Jones MM, Fortney SM. Saline ingestion during lower body negative pressure as an end-of-mission countermeasure to post-space flight orthostatic intolerance. 43rd Congress of International Astronautical Federation, IAF/IAA-92-0267, 1992
9. West JB, Guy HJB, Elliott AR et al. Respiratory system in microgravity In: Handbook of physiology. Section 4: Environmental physiology. Volume I. Fregly MJ, Blatteis CM (eds). Oxford: Oxford University Press, 1996:675-688
10. Guy HJB, Prisk GK, Elliott AR et al. Inequality of pulmonary ventilation during sustained microgravity as determined from single-breath washouts. J Appl Physiol (Respiration Environmental Exerc Physiol) 1994; 76:1719-1729
11. Daunton NG. Adaptation of the vestibular system to microgravity In: Handbook of physiology. Section 4: Environmental physiology. Volume I. Fregly MJ, Blatteis CM (eds). Oxford: Oxford University Press, 1996:765-783
12. Vernikos J. Human physiology in space. Bioessays 1996; 18:1029-1037
13. Reschke MF, Bloomberg JJ, Harm DL et al. Posture, locomotion, spatial orientation and motion sickness as a function of space flight [Short review]. Brain Res Reviews 1998; 28:102-117
14. Roll R, Gilhodes JC, Roll JP et al. Proprioceptive information processing in weightlessness. Exper Brain Res 1998; 122:393-402
15. Edgerton VR, Roy RR. Neuromuscular adaptations to actual and simulated spaceflight. In: Handbook of physiology. Section 4: Environmental physiology. Volume I. Fregly MJ, Blatteis CM (eds). Oxford: Oxford University Press, 1996:721-763
16. Widrick JJ, Knuth ST, Norenberg KM et al. Effect of a 17 day spaceflight on contractile properties of human soleus muscle fibres. J Physiol 1999; 516:915-930
17. Morey-Holton ER, Whalen RT, Arnaud SB et al. The skeleton and its adaptation to gravity. In: Handbook of physiology. Section 4: Environmental physiology. Volume I. Fregly MJ, Blatteis CM (eds). Oxford: Oxford University Press, 1996:691-719

18. Caillot-Augusseau A, Lafage-Proust MH, Soler C et al. Bone formation and resorption biological markers in cosmonauts during and after a 180-day space flight (Euromir 95). Clin Chem 1998; 44:578-585

19. Biklc DD, Halloran BP. The response of bone to unloading. J Bone Miner Metab 1999; 17:233-244

20. Inoue M, Tanaka H, Moriwake T et al. Altered biochemical markers of bone turnover in humans during 120 days of bed rest. Bone 2000; 26:281-286

21. McCarthy I, Goodship A, Herzog R et al. Investigation of bone changes in microgravity during long and short duration space flight: comparison of techniques. Europ J Clin Inv 2000; 30:1044-1054

22. Loomer PM. The impact of microgravity on bone metabolism in vitro and in vivo. Crit Rev Oral Biol Med 2001; 12:252-261

23. Zittermann A, Heer M, Caillot-Augusso A et al. Microgravity inhibits intestinal calcium absorption as shown by a stable strontium test. Europ J Clin Inv 2000; 30:1036-1043

24. Borchers AT, Keen CL, Gershwin ME. Microgravity and immune responsiveness: implications for space travel. Nutrition 2002; 18:889-898

25. Sonnenfeld G, Shearer WT. Immune function during space flight. Nutrition, 2002; 18:899-903

26. Homick JL, Reschke MF. Postural equilibrium following exposure to weightless space flight. Acta Otolaryngol 1977; 83:455-464

27. Arbeille P, Achaïbou F, Fomina G et al. Regional blood flow in microgravity: adaptation and deconditioning. Med Sci Sports Exerc 1996; 28:S70-S79

28. Baisch FJ, Wolfram G, Beck L et al. Orthostatic stress is necessary to maintain the dynamic range of cardiovascular control in space. Pflugers Archiv 2000; 441:R52-R61

29. Convertino VA. Planning strategies for development of effective exercise and nutrition countermeasures for long-duration space flight. Nutrition 2002; 18:880-888

30. Heer M, Boerger A, Kamps N et al. Nutrient supply during recent European missions. Pflugers Archiv 2000; 441:R8-R14

31. Heer M, Kamps N, Biener C et al. Calcium metabolism in microgravity. Europ J Med Res 1999; 4:357-360.

Chapter 8

Air quality

CHAPTER CONTENTS

Introduction 145
Primary pollutants 146
Secondary pollutants 153

The human factor 156
Ionization and antigens 158
Overview 160

INTRODUCTION

The developed economies have been characterized by movements of their populations from rural to urban areas. Such migration has been linked with better employment opportunities in the towns and cities. There has been increased reliance on the use of energy sources to sustain both industrial and domestic requirements. Industrial developments have often been at a cost of reducing the purity of environmental air, polluting soil and water with potential adverse effects on the food-chain. The concern about environmental pollution is now global, as a result of serious accidents in the nuclear industry, and oil and water pollution, and there is a recognition of the delicate ecological balance in nature.

Utilization of energy is the main underlying source of air pollutants. Many chemicals are added to the ambient air each day as a result of industrial processes, motor vehicle traffic and the use of energy for domestic and recreational purposes. Environmental factors may interact with prevailing pollution levels to accentuate the discomfort of individuals exposed. There is concern, especially among factory-based occupational physicians, that pollutants may be detrimental to health. Various pollutants have also been studied with regard to their effects during the performance of exercise, whether in competitive training or recreational contexts. There is also interest in how pristine air might be used to enhance mood and well-being.

The purity of ambient air is thought to be a very important component of so-called quality of life. The expansion in size of Buenos Aires, the capital city of Argentina, was linked with its reputation for good air and explains its name. Ironically, the growth of large conurbations has been a cause of impairing air quality due to a variety of reasons including industrial processes and motor vehicle traffic. Yet air pollution is not a feature of urban environments only, since polluted air may be blown into rural areas to hover over rural valleys between adjacent mountains. The worst pollution in Scotland is found not in the cities of Edinburgh or Glasgow but in the sparsely populated Highlands.

Pollutants can be classified as primary or secondary, depending on whether they retain the form in which they were emitted from source when their effects are realized or if they are formed through chemical reactions between source and target. Among the primary pollutants are sulphur dioxide (SO_2), carbon monoxide (CO), nitrogen oxides especially nitrogen dioxide (NO_2), benzene and particulate matter like dust and smoke. Particulates less than 10 microns in diameter are referred to as PM-10s.

The secondary pollutants ozone (O_3) and peroxyacetyl nitrate (PAN) are formed by means of the effects of ultraviolet radiation on the primary pollutants nitrogen dioxide and hydrocarbons. Ozone is formed by a reaction cycle involving nitrogen monoxide, nitrogen dioxide, oxygen, hydrocarbons and energy from ultraviolet radiation. Photochemical oxidant refers to the pollutant mixture generated in this process, exemplified by the photochemical smog in the Los Angeles Basin. The oxidant pollutant family includes ozone, oxides of nitrogen (NO_x) and the hydrocarbons. Acid fog refers to the formation of sulphuric acid in dilute solution when SO_2 is present with a high moisture content in the air.

Primary pollutants are considered in this chapter before attention is directed towards secondary pollutants, typically in outdoor settings. Indoor pollutants are then reviewed before protective mechanisms and mitigating factors are addressed. There is also consideration given to the effects of air ionization on mood states and their implications for human performance.

PRIMARY POLLUTANTS

Sulphur dioxide

Burning carbon fuels such as soft coals produces particles of sulphur dioxide (SO_2) and the more toxic sulphur trioxide (SO_3). Sulphur dioxide is circulated in the air from local smoke stacks that generate unwanted smog. This pollutant is produced by smelters, refineries and electrical utilities that use fossil fuels to generate energy. It is the primary pollutant involved in the formation of acidic aerosols and in some developing countries, notably in Asia, can reach levels high enough to impair lung function and exercise performance in healthy individuals.

Sulphur dioxide, like ozone, is an airway irritant with potential harmful effects on the epithelial cells lining the airways and alveoli. It may also cause changes in mucous secretions and mucociliary clearance. The effects depend in the main on the pollutant dose delivered to the lung. It is a highly soluble gas and tends to be removed by the moist surfaces of the nose and upper airways. A blocked nose, due to a cold or an allergic reaction, or participation in exercise will cause a shift to breathing through the mouth which has a poorer 'scrubbing' capacity. In these cases the gas is likely to reach the intrathoracic airways and, in high doses, affect lung function.

Sulphur dioxide is a more common pollutant than ozone but at equivalent concentrations has far less impact on lung function. Its threshold level for affecting pulmonary function in healthy individuals has been estimated to be between 1 and 2 ppm,[1] a value that is 5-10 times higher than that for ozone. At current ambient levels it is unlikely that endurance exercise will be affected in normal healthy individuals. Asthmatics exposed to concentrations of 0.25 ppm while exercising for 2-10 minutes may have their symptoms worsened. Wheezing, dyspnoea and chest tightness may result and require the use of a bronchodilator.[2] Two-fold increases in airway resistance have been reported in asthmatics exercising for five minutes with SO_2 concentrations around 0.5 ppm. Repeated exposures within the same day induce a much less severe response.[3]

Sulphur dioxide inhaled with cold dry air induces bronchoconstriction at concentrations of 0.25 ppm, or, at higher concentrations, worsens the effects of bronchoconstriction.[1] Effects are not noted in all asthmatics as there is a large range of sensitivity to SO_2. Bronchoconstriction caused by SO_2 can be inhibited by prior administration of cromolyn sodium.[4] Use of β2-agonist medication, such as salbutamol, can relieve symptoms and reverse the adverse effects on lung function. Theoretically, a combination of SO_2 and O_3 would be expected to yield addictive effects on pulmonary function but experimental support for the additive impact is lacking.[5]

Carbon monoxide

Emissions of carbon monoxide (CO) in the atmosphere are greater than those of all other air pollutants combined. Carbon monoxide pollution is especially prevalent in urban environments. Urban levels of CO are derived largely from combustion of fossil fuels and other carbonaceous materials like coal, mineral oils, wood and tobacco. Undefined natural processes of removal prevent the background level of CO rising year on year.

Motor vehicle exhaust fumes are the primary source of CO in urban air. Carbon monoxide is toxic and is not easily detected by human senses. It is a common cause of accidental death during sleep and is used as a painless means of suicide inside a car, by connecting the exhaust pipe to the car's interior.

The affinity of haemoglobin for CO is over 200 times that for oxygen and so inhaled CO is easily taken up by the bloodstream. The consequence is a reduction in the oxygen carrying capacity of the blood. Carbon monoxide

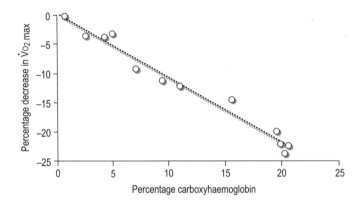

Figure 8.1 The effect of increasing carboxyhaemoglobin level on maximal oxygen uptake in healthy participants. After Folinsbee LJ, Schelegle ES. Air pollutants and endurance performance[2]

attaches to the haemoglobin in red blood cells to form carboxyhaemoglobin (COHb). Performance of endurance exercise is likely to be affected as a result of a reduction in the O_2 delivered to the active muscles. If COHb levels increase to 20%, clinical symptoms of CO poisoning are observed.[1] The strong attraction of Hb for CO is due to the haemoglobin molecule's scavenging function of preventing a build-up of CO in the body arising from the breakdown of red blood cells. The elimination of CO through the lungs is therefore an innate protective mechanism.

Carbon monoxide is one of the 2000 or so chemicals produced as a result of cigarette smoking. Consequently, the oxygen transport capacity of smokers is reduced and there is also a partial effect associated with passive smoking. The normal COHb level in non-smokers' blood is 0.5 to 0.7%, whereas values ten times greater may be observed in frequent smokers. The normal value in non-smokers can be increased five-fold in city dwellers. In urban areas, ambient CO levels can range from 15 to 100 ppm and their impact depends on the duration of exposure and the individual's minute ventilation ($\dot{V}E$), both factors raising the concentrations of COHb.

The maximal oxygen uptake ($\dot{V}O_{2\,max}$) is reduced in a linear fashion as the COHb concentrations in blood increase (see Figure 8.1). Carboxyhaemoglobin levels of less than 4% have no effect on maximal oxygen uptake but a value of 15% or more causes a corresponding 15% reduction in $\dot{V}O_{2\,max}$ and an increase of 2 beats min⁻¹ in maximal heart rate; at this exposure level there is a 19% increase in $\dot{V}E$ response to sub-maximal exercise.[1] In this study by Follinsbee et al., the $\dot{V}O_{2\,max}$ at 20% COHb declined by 24% but there was no further change in maximal heart rate; the ventilatory response to sub-maximal exercise was elevated by 33%. The maximal cardiac output was not affected, indicating that the decrease in $\dot{V}O_{2\,max}$ was attributable to a reduction in oxygen transport, some of the oxygen in arterial blood being replaced by carbon monoxide. The decrease in oxygen carrying capacity of the blood is compensated for at sub-maximal exercise by an increased cardiac output. The rise in minute ventilation during sub-maximal exercise is analogous to responses to altitude hypoxia when, despite the changes in pulmonary function, the oxygen uptake is unaltered. The difference is that the haemoglobin saturation is reduced at altitude whereas CO reduces the number of sites available for transporting oxygen around the circulation.

Endurance exercise can be adversely affected by a rise in COHb before any fall in $\dot{V}O_{2\,max}$ is apparent. Folinsbee, Horvath and Raven[1] referred to a series of studies by their own research groups in which subjects exercised to maximum whilst breathing air containing 50, 75 and 100 ppm CO. Exercise time to exhaustion was decreased when the COHb levels of non-smokers reached 2.7%, but $\dot{V}O_{2\,max}$ did not decrease until values reached 4.3%. These findings have consequences for performance in endurance sports such as road running and field games where competitors engage 70-80% of their maximal aerobic power output. At low exercise intensities in the range 30-60% $\dot{V}O_{2\,max}$, there may be little or no adverse effect since ambient levels of CO leading to COHb concentrations less than 15% do not increase the physiological responses in healthy subjects. It is possible, however, that cognitive functions are adversely affected once blood COHb levels exceed 5%. At exercise intensities of 65-85% $\dot{V}O_{2\,max}$, the capability to sustain endurance exercise may be impaired, the cardiac output being no longer able to compensate for the decreased oxygen carrying capacity of the blood when COHb is 3-5%. Elevation of COHb can alter the 'lactate threshold', causing an increase in ventilation and blood lactate and a decrease in end-tidal CO_2 when exercise intensity exceeds this threshold.[6]

Carbon monoxide levels are likely to be raised near motorways with heavy traffic. Thus pollution could be a nuisance to cyclists and distance runners who use the public road for training purposes. Both groups tend to avoid racing immediately behind mechanically propelled vehicles and so do not incur large doses of this pollutant. When ambient levels of CO are below 6 ppm, COHb levels do not rise. Joggers in ambient levels of CO exceeding 7 ppm begin to accumulate CO in their bodies.[7] Therefore the relationship between CO and the associated biological burden is not linear.

Portable CO monitors that were attached to the bicycles of commuters in Boston, USA, recorded average exposures of up to 17 ppm, and peak levels of CO over 100 ppm were recorded on urban highways in the 1970s. This research preceded the widespread introduction of exhaust catalysts. Anderson et al.[8] found that very light exercise (walking) along a busy road increased COHb levels by 1% and Nicholson and Case[9] reported that 30 minutes of jogging in urban New York increased COHb levels to 5.1%, a level characteristic of heavy smokers and one that would be expected to hinder athletic performance. Waldman et al.[10] compared the effects of cycling to driving a car during rush hours in Washington DC on COHb levels. The cyclists' levels rose by only 0.9% compared to the 2.1% rise in the motorists. These results were surprising since ambient CO levels were above 60 ppm on

11 of the 29 days that the study lasted and the cyclists did not show any detrimental changes in pulmonary function or time to exhaustion on a treadmill run after their journey. An increased incidence of eye irritation was reported by the cyclists. Atkinson[11] suggested that cyclists may, unlike a motorist, be able to move to the front of a traffic queue, thus avoiding direct exposure to exhaust emissions; the CO concentration at the end of a car exhaust is about 20,000 ppm. The cyclists studied by Waldman and co-workers[10] were not performing *intense* exercise but merely commuting in the city, and competitive cyclists with high ventilation volumes are likely to be more affected.

Air pollutants including CO may enter the tanks of a sports diver (scuba), during filling, either from vehicle emissions in urban air or from the compressor that is used in filling the tanks. Contaminated air may become a special problem during deep dives since the partial pressures of all the inspired gases are greatly increased.

In mountaineering and other outdoor sports, gas and petrol stoves are used to cook food. Individuals must be careful when using these stoves inside tents or snow holes since CO levels can increase rapidly due to incomplete combustion. Gill[12] recorded levels of CO of up to 300 ppm in such environments. These ambient levels can result in COHb concentration of 10% which is high enough to hinder the performance of these individuals or, if combined with the environmental stress of altitude, to exacerbate the symptoms of acute mountain sickness.[13]

Travelling by car for several hours along polluted roads may expose athletes to pollutants even before competition takes place. Aranow et al.[14] reported a mean COHb level of 5.1% in subjects who drove along a motorway. A smoker present in the car accentuates the problem and the fact that the half-life for CO removal can be four hours does make matters worse.[15] Results from Atkinson and Tindall[16] indicated that 30 minutes of exercise at 70% $\dot{V}O_{2\,max}$ does not accelerate the elimination of smoking-induced CO from the body, a finding applicable to other sources of CO inhalation. Swimmers travelling by car through polluted urban areas prior to competition experienced negative effects on performance.[17] Since these studies were conducted, the adverse effects of CO have been recognised by motor vehicle manufacturers and modern vehicles have lower emissions of this harmful gas.

Nitrogen oxides

Nitrogen oxides constitute a family of highly reactive gases emanating mainly from motor vehicle exhaust and electrical utilities. Since they are needed, along with sunlight and volatile organic compounds, to generate ozone, their ambient concentrations fall as ozone is produced photochemically. Nitrogen dioxide (NO_2) is the most likely member of this family of gases to affect lung function, but the high concentrations that would cause serious concern are rarely recorded in normal ambient environments. It has a potentiating effect in the presence of ozone;[18] pre-exposure to 0.6 ppm

NO_2 accentuated the impairment in lung function caused by 0.3 ppm ozone. Nevertheless, on its own and at exposure levels of 0.5 ppm, NO_2 caused a decrease in resistance to respiratory infection.[19] Nitrogen oxides also generate free radicals in the lungs and cause inflammation as a consequence.[20]

Indoor ice-skating arenas are the most important source of nitrogen dioxide emission in a sports environment. Skating rinks engage mechanics to resurface, clean and smooth the ice during an operating day. Typically, the machines are powered by petrol or propane. They can emit too much CO and NO_2 into the ice rink and these gases then accumulate in its enclosed space, depending on how well the rink is maintained. There is a long history of pollutant-related illness recorded amongst ice-rink specialists. Poisoning from nitrogen dioxide has been reported in ice-hockey players[21] and ice-hockey referees.[22] There have also been suggestions that toxic substances associated with the cleaning of ice rinks have been linked with menstrual irregularities in elite figure skaters.[23]

The median indoor NO_2 concentration in seventy ice rinks in the USA was found to be 180 ppb.[24] Weekly averages exceeding 1000 ppb were reported for 10% of the rinks. Serious CO intoxication has also been reported in ice- hockey players, ice rink technicians and figure skaters.[11] It would seem important, therefore, that the quality of the air should be monitored regularly in ice rinks.

Atkinson[11] reported maximum hourly concentrations of NO_2 in urban areas were 43-271 ppb during 1993. These figures compare with the hourly limit of 210 ppb set by the World Health Organisation, which was exceeded on only one day during the year. Concentrations in rural areas were 15-54 ppb, so this pollutant is not a major concern away from the cities.

Benzene

Benzene is an aromatic hydrocarbon (C_6H_6). It is a colourless liquid obtained from coal tar oil and is used as a source of fuel for mechanically propelled vehicles. Its concentrations in the atmosphere have increased in recent years whereas, due to governmental controls, lead levels from motor engine combustion are decreasing.

Atkinson[11] reported maximum concentrations of 0.7 to 1.4 ppb in urban areas in the United Kingdom, calculated as a rolling average throughout 1993. The standard recommended by the Environmental Protection Agency was 5 ppb (annual rolling mean). A longer-term standard of 1 ppb has also been recommended.

Few studies have been undertaken on the biological burden of environmental benzene levels. Likewise, the impact of these levels on health and exercise performance has not been investigated extensively.

Lead

Environmental levels of lead have decreased since the introduction of unleaded petrol in motor vehicles. In countries where lead is still added to petrol, lead particles are emitted from vehicular exhaust fumes into the air. Lead levels in the United Kingdom decreased seven-fold between 1980 and 1993. In the latter years annual mean concentrations were 78-147 ng.m^{-3} in urban areas and 8-37 ng.m^{-3} in rural areas.

In the early 1990s, Atkinson et al.[25] studied the blood lead levels of cyclists competing and habitually training on dual-carriageway motorways in the north east of England. The expectation was that those training in areas likely to be polluted would experience increased biological doses of lead. Although significant relationships were found between the cyclists' blood lead levels and their training characteristics, the lead absorption of about 0.5 μmol/l was no higher than that of the sedentary subjects. This observation suggested the cyclists were not carrying any burden associated with elevated blood lead concentrations although those who specialized in time trial events showed blood lead levels 0.2 μmol/l higher than that of sedentary subjects. The time triallists displayed blood lead levels 0.2 μmol/l higher after a race held on a dual carriageway than a road-racing group whose competition was in a rural area. These differences could not have been due to any exercise-induced effects since they were not observed in a laboratory with a constant ambient concentration of lead. All the blood lead levels recorded in the study complied with European Union regulations regarding lead exposure.

Athletes absorb significant amounts of lead when lead concentrations in the air are high, a view supported by the results of studies carried out in the Republic of South Africa. Up to 1989, there was 0.6-0.8 g of lead added to petrol in South Africa which is similar to additions to British petrol in the 1970s. Extremely high blood lead levels (mean 2.5 μmol/l) in athletes who trained in urban areas were reported by van Rensburg et al.[26] and Grobler et al.[27] Such levels would be expected to mediate several detrimental effects on haemostasis and nervous system function. Grant-White[28] suggested that lead absorption and the associated influence on the brain and behaviour may adequately explain the phenomenon of running addiction or what he explained as 'marathon mania'. No material evidence for this speculative link was provided. Grobler et al.[29] re-examined the blood lead levels of South African runners after the 1989 reduction in petrol lead and found the degree of lead absorption had dropped markedly in urban-training athletes to about 0.8 μmol/l. There was no accompanying measurement of so-called running addiction for which habituation to elevations in brain endorphins has been presented as explanation.

Competitive shooting in indoor firing ranges can cause the production of lead oxide fumes by the combustion of the printing compounds and fragmentation of the bullet when fired. Serious lead poisoning has been reported in instructors at an indoor pistol range. The blood lead levels of these subjects were above 5 μmol/l. Stromme et al.[30] reported that 43% of a sample of Norwegian pistol shooters had blood lead levels exceeding 1.5 μmol/l, while 22% exhibited levels between 2.0 and 2.7 μmol/l. A control group was not examined in this study. A very precise analytical technique is required to assess lead levels in blood, especially to ensure samples are not contaminated.

PM-10s

Particulate matter which is less than 10 μm is referred to by the abbreviation PM-10. These particles are small enough to reach the lower areas of the respiratory tract. Levels of PM-10s have increased in recent years, particularly by the sides of busy roadways. There has not been a corresponding increase in research into the effects of PM-10s on exercise performance.

Levels of PM-10s may also be high at indoor sports arenas. Georghiou et al.[31] reported a positive correlation between the number of spectators smoking at an ice arena and the air levels of PM-10. It is important therefore to consider the banning of smoking at such events for health as well as safety reasons. Smoking in domestic circumstances can also have a negative impact, as home-based tobacco smoke was found to impair ventilatory function and retard lung development in children.[32]

The maximum hourly concentrations of PM-10s in urban areas of the United Kingdom were 76-445 μg.m^{-3} in 1993. In most British cities, the 50 μg.m^{-3} regulatory standard is regularly exceeded. Adverse effects on health result from inflammation mediated by oxidative stress.[33] Asthmatic individuals and people with cardiovascular disease are especially at risk when PM-10s rise above the regulatory limit.

SECONDARY POLLUTANTS

Ozone

The formation of ozone (O_3) is the result of a reaction cycle that involves nitrogen monoxide, nitrogen dioxide, oxygen, hydrocarbons and energy from ultraviolet radiation. Like sulphur dioxide, ozone is a major airway irritant. Ozone causes irritation to the airways in resting and moderately exercising individuals at concentrations of 0.30 ppm. When the high ventilation volumes of elite athletes are considered, the airway constrictive effect of ozone is evident at concentrations as low as 0.20 ppm.[1] Ozone causes breathing rates to increase and tidal volume to decrease at a given exercise intensity and these changes are accompanied by substernal pain.

Ozone exerts much of its clinical effects by means of irritating the airways. It can also damage epithelial cells lining airways and alveoli, and affect mucous secretions and functioning of the cilia. Damage to the epithelial cells triggers an increase in inflammatory neutrophils. High ozone concentrations cause tracheal irritation, and decrease diffusing capacity and maximum expiratory flow. The lungs' antioxidant defences are able to deal with low ozone doses even in sustained exposure but can be overwhelmed by short exposures to higher doses. At concentrations above 1 ppm, ozone can lead to pulmonary oedema and ultimately death. The air quality standard in the USA states that ozone levels shall not exceed 0.12 ppm (based on a one-hour averaging time) more than once per annum. In the United Kingdom the 8-hourly 0.05 ppm limit was exceeded on 0-11 days (urban) and 0-39 days (rural) over one year.[11]

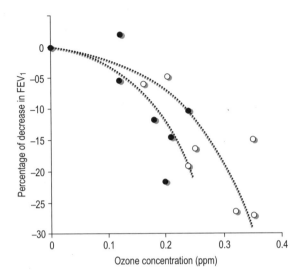

Figure 8.2 The relative decline in lung function after 60 min continuous exercise on exposure to 0.12- 0.35 ppm ozone. Responses were estimated for two exercise intensities corresponding to minute ventilation rates of 60-70 l/min (○) and 80-100 l/min (●)

In the USA the Environmental Protection Agency issues a 'first stage alert' or health advisory notice when ozone levels exceed 0.20 ppm. A 'second stage alert' is issued when ozone levels go above 0.35 ppm. An endurance athlete's performance is unlikely to be affected by prior exposure at rest to ozone unless the levels exceed the second stage alert standard.[34]

Ozone concentrations in the range 0.12-0.18 ppm cause significant symptoms and decrements in pulmonary function when exercise of moderate intensity is sustained for 60 minutes.[2] This result occurs irrespective of whether the exercise is continuous or an intermittent protocol (see Figure 8.2). When exercise was continued for longer than this time, trained cyclists suffered respiratory symptoms and small decrements in lung function, at ozone levels below 0.09 ppm.[35]

There was considerable research interest in the potential consequences of exposure to ozone in the years prior to the 1984 Los Angeles Olympic Games. In the Los Angeles Basin, peak levels typically occur around midday but could persist for some hours, depending on prevailing meteorological conditions. Athletes engaged in heavy exercise for 30 minutes or more could experience functional or symptomatic respiratory problems at concentrations as low as 0.15-0.20 ppm. Such levels occur frequently at the inland sites of the Los Angeles area and are expected on 50% of the days in July and August. The Olympic events were scheduled to avoid the midday peak ozone levels, which were predicted to be lower at the competition sites closer to the shore. In the event, photochemical air pollution was uncharacteristically low, and so it was not possible to establish relationships between ambient air pollution and performance of elite athletes in field circumstances.

Reports of the effects of ambient air pollutants on athletes exercising outdoors have been limited. One study conducted in a section of the Los Angeles Basin with especially poor air quality showed a decrease in FVC following two-hour outdoor American football practices at the first stage alert level (0.20 ppm O_3) and higher.[15] Prior to this, a group of high school cross-country runners had been studied[36] over a period of six years to determine if there was a relationship between poor running performance, which was defined as a failure to improve race times as the season progressed, and the oxidant pollution levels one hour prior to the race. The winner required only 12 minutes to run the race, so results may not apply to events lasting longer than this time. When the oxidant level exceeded 0.25 ppm, as many as 50% of the members of the team had a decreased running performance. In contrast, when the oxidant level was below 0.10 ppm, fewer than 20% of the team members had decreased performance.

A less than maximal effort due to discomfort from inhaling ozone may be the cause of the decreased performance, rather than a true physiological impairment of the oxygen transport mechanism. A rise in ambient ozone levels is typically associated with increased ambient temperature, primarily because of the temperature inversion and stagnant air that produces a pollution episode. The effect of the combined heat and ozone may be difficult to differentiate. Early experimental studies of combined heat and ozone exposure[1] showed an additive effect on lung function changes, i.e. both stresses are associated with diminished performance on lung function tests. Thus, it may often be difficult to differentiate the performance effects due to heat exposure from those due to air pollution.

Following repeated exposure to ozone, there is a period of decreased responsiveness to the acute effects of ozone, a phenomenon which has been termed 'adaptation'. This terminology has been criticised for a number of reasons and Follinsbee, Horvath and Raven[1] preferred the term 'desensitisation'. Hackney et al.[37] provided the initial evidence that residents of polluted areas may be less sensitive to ozone than those who live in more pristine air environments. Students newly arrived in Los Angeles were compared with a similar group of students who were residents of Los Angeles. The newcomers were slightly more sensitive to the effects of ozone on pulmonary function than were the residents. Hackney et al.[38] also compared a group from eastern Canada with a Los Angeles group; again, the non-resident group was somewhat more sensitive to ozone.

Follinsbee, Horvath and Raven[39] concluded that repeated ambient exposure over several weeks or months would induce what they termed an adaptation to ozone. Pre-exposure for 2 or 3 days to the polluted environment in which the competitive event is to occur may provide such a so-called adaptation that would enable the performer to exercise without physiological impairment.

The prospect of ozone affecting the performance of athletes was also a major concern prior to the 2004 Summer Olympics in Athens. The city itself is situated in a basin that is open to the sea on one side and is surrounded by mountains on the other three sides. Industrial emissions in both the basin and the neighbouring plain combine with unfavourable meteorological and topographical conditions to produce relatively high pollution levels in the air. Sea breezes stratify the atmosphere directly above the city so that the polluted air is trapped between the mountains and remains at a low altitude. Offshore breezes waft the air towards the sea in the evenings but the onshore breeze during the day recirculates the pollutants back into the basin. The main pollutants are the photochemical oxidants, oxides of nitrogen and ozone. A programme of incentives for motorists led to a decrease in the former pollutant in the city centre and the latter in the outskirts.[40] As in Los Angeles 20 years earlier, the likely effects on athletes were difficult to predict because of the distribution of competitive sites, the climatic conditions to be encountered and the fact that very few relevant studies had been conducted on elite athletes.

Peroxyacetyl nitrate

Peroxyacetyl nitrate (PAN) is another secondary product of photochemical oxidation. Its concentration in the air is rarely above 0.1 ppm. Its main effect seems to be an irritant to the eyes but its symptoms can also include blurred vision and eye fatigue.[41]

Prolonged exercise has no significant effect on cardiovascular or pulmonary function at exposures to 0.24 ppm PAN. Exposure over four hours led to a 4% decline in forced vital capacity which was attributed to slight decreases in inspiratory capacity and in expiratory reserve volume.[42] Shorter exercise periods with subjects exposed to the same level of PAN did not cause any significant changes in lung function. Any effect on performance may be attributable to the discomfort due to irritation of the eyes. Younger men appear to be more affected than are older men, but the existence of any gender effect has not been experimentally studied.

THE HUMAN FACTOR

Human characteristics

Laboratory-based studies of human responses to various pollutants have led to a number of generalisations. The major conclusions are as follows:

- The concentration of pollutants in inspired air or in the blood is negatively related to pulmonary ventilation. Ultimately there is a consequent impact on exercise performance
- There is individual sensitivity to effects of air pollution
- The detrimental effects of air pollutants are accentuated in asthmatic individuals.

Athletes are particularly at risk from inhaling air pollutants for a number of reasons, including:

- Ventilation (the $\dot{V}E$) is increased progressively with the exercise intensity and there is a corresponding rise in the amount of pollutants inhaled
- The increase in airflow velocity transports pollutants further into the respiratory passages
- More air is inhaled through oral breathing during exercise and less through the nose, so that the normal nasal mechanisms for filtering out large particles and soluble vapours are bypassed.

Another line of defence for the body is the trapping, transport and scrubbing of pollutants by the mucosal surfaces and cilia of the tracheobronchial tree. There is evidence that after exercise in an urban context, mucociliary action is impaired for several days.[43] It is thought that athletes experience an increased susceptibility to upper respiratory tract infections during these days.

Preventive measures

McCafferty[15] recommended that exercise is avoided when pollutant concentrations exceed air quality standards, that training should be scheduled at times associated with the least air pollution, that urban-based athletes should choose less congested training routes, and that athletes should travel to competitions well before start-time with the car windows closed, and in a vehicle free of tobacco smoke. It would be prudent to train hardest in the evening after pollution levels fall and the body's circadian rhythms are amenable to tolerating high-intensity exercise.[44]

Activated carbon face-masks are sometimes used by athletes training in urban environments. These masks probably increase the energy cost of ventilation during intense exercise, are only partially effective and do not protect against all gaseous pollutants. Besides, they should have the filters changed frequently for effective removal of particulates.

Controlling the pollutant exposure of indoor sports competitors is more difficult than with outdoor recreation. Improvements in ventilation appear to improve air quality in indoor pistol firing ranges.[45] Bauer et al.[46] maintained that the use of an extended exhaust pipe on an ice-resurfacer, limiting the number of hours of operation of the machine, or improving rink ventilation were individually ineffective in reducing pollution in an ice arena to acceptable limits. Lee et al.[19] recommended that all the above modifications be made in combination and suggested that ice arenas switch to using battery-powered ice maintenance machines as a more acceptable alternative.

There have been suggestions that some protection against the adverse physiological effects of ozone is obtained as a result of ingesting antioxidant substances. In particular, vitamin C and vitamin E would fulfil this role. There has been some evidence of a positive effect of these vitamins in countering adverse effects of oxidant agents. Samet et al.[47] found that 250 mg of vitamin C attenuated the decrement in lung function induced by 0.4 ppm ozone in individuals exercising at moderate intensity. Grievink et al.[35] reported the similarly positive effects of providing cyclists with a supplement mixture of 100 mg vitamin E and 500 mg vitamin C daily for 15 weeks. Some of the effects of ozone can be mitigated by cyclo-oxygenase inhibitors[2] whilst inhaled beta-agonists can reverse ozone-induced bronchoconstriction in asthmatics.

IONIZATION AND ANTIGENS

Air ions

Air ions may be produced in nature by events such as the shearing of water droplets in a waterfall and the rapid flow of great volumes of air over a land mass, and by solar and cosmic radiation, as well as by a variety of radioactive sources. The ions are produced by these sources of energy that displace an electron from a molecule of one of the common atmospheric gases. The molecule is left with a positive charge whilst the displaced electron is normally captured by another molecule to which it imparts a negative charge.

Air ions are generally recognised as biologically active. Negative air ions are thought to promote beneficial mood states whilst positive air ions have been shown to cause characteristic complaints from subjects.[48] Accordingly, negative air ion generators are commercially available for office and domestic environments to enhance mood and performance. Hawkins and Barker[47] reported experimental evidence that negative air ions produced positive effects on psychomotor and mental functions.

Favourable effects may also extend to conditions of physical exercise. Sovijarvi et al.[49] showed that perceived exertion during an incremental exercise test was lowered by an excess of negative air ions compared to a condition of excess positive ions. This finding was supported by Inbar et al.[50] who reported that the elevation in heart rate and core temperature during exercise was less pronounced on exposure to negative air ions compared with neutral air.

The mechanisms through which the effects of air ions are mediated may include brain levels of serotonin,[51] body temperature[52] and oxidative metabolism.[53] All of these functions vary with the 24-hour solar day and so exposure to air ions may disturb normal circadian rhythms. Hawkins and Barker[48] reported that subjects exposed to negative air ions demonstrated a flattening of the normal curve in performance (mirror tracking, reaction time and pursuit rotor test); in contrast, performance on exposure to positive air ions showed an exaggerated decline in the evening compared to a control condition.

Reilly and Stevenson[54] confirmed that negative air ions produce biological effects since significant reductions were found in rectal temperature, heart rate and metabolic rate at rest on exposure to negative air ionization. The reduction in temperature was attributed to a drop in metabolic rate rather than a direct effect on thermoregulatory mechanisms. It has been shown *in vitro* that large doses of negative air ions promote the efficiency of aerobic and metabolic processes.[51,53] This effect could partly account for the decreases at rest in $\dot{V}O_2$ and $\dot{V}E$ and, consequently, in heart rate noted by Reilly and Stevenson.[53] Additionally, Inbar et al.[50] have suggested that coupling of electron transport and ATP synthesis is more efficient under the influence of small negative air ions, causing less liberation of heat energy. However, the changes in $\dot{V}O_2$ due to air ionization reported by Reilly and Stevenson[54] were comparatively greater than those in body temperature. They concluded that factors other than thermoregulatory mechanisms mediate the influence of air ions on tissue metabolism. The effects observed on metabolism and heart rate at rest tended to disappear under exercise conditions. Sovijarvi et al.[49] found benefits to persist during exercise, noting a tendency towards lower heart rates and decreased ratings of exertion on exposure to negative air ions compared with exposure to positive air ions. The effects may be subject-specific, since individual variability in responsiveness to air was shown by Charry,[54] using reaction time as a criterion.

The effect of negative air ions on rectal temperature evident at rest was found to persist under sub-maximal exercise intensities.[53] The difference of 0.2°C was small and of little practical significance for light levels of exercise. However, the effect could have important implications for conditions when thermoregulatory requirements place limits on exercise performance.[55] This would apply at high intensities and longer durations of exercise, when thermoregulatory mechanisms are severely challenged. The normal timing of circadian rhythms in body temperature and metabolism[57] is unaffected by air ions but the amplitude is reduced. It would also be relevant when heavy physical work has to be sustained in hot environments.

The flattening of the curve in body temperature caused by exposure to negative air ions supports the hypothesis of Hawkins and Barker[48] whose views were based on performance rhythms. It is well known that performance in many psychomotor tasks follows the normal circadian curve in body temperature. To what extent the effects of air ions on the body temperature rhythms and performance rhythms noted by Hawkins and Barker[48] are due to common mechanisms is not easily established. The suggestion was that the effect may be mediated by brain serotonin levels which are known to be influenced by air ions and are implicated also in the central neural control of circadian rhythms.[58]

Observations of Reilly and Stevenson[54] confirmed that negative air ions are biologically active but their effects are diminished when physiological responses to exercise are considered. The effect on rectal temperature, though small in magnitude, still persisted during exercise. Nevertheless, it is not clear how the reduction in core temperature in itself is related to the improved mood and positive disposition towards exercise performance. The amplitude of the normal circadian rhythms was reduced from 0.27 to 0.15°C on exposure to negative air ions. This observation is difficult to interpret, although the finding may have implications for the use of ion therapy in the period of transition after crossing multiple time-zones or when moving onto nocturnal work shifts.

Allergens

Allergens such as pollens or house dust alight first in the nose where they are filtered out. Allergic reactions of the airways first begin in the nose. The resulting inflammatory response caused by mast-cell discharge blocks the nose and leads to a shift towards breathing through the mouth. As a consequence, the allergens achieve direct access to the lower respiratory tract where an inflammatory response can now trigger an asthma attack. Allergens from different flora may also cause allergic reactions leading to irritation of mucous membranes of the eye as well as of those of the respiratory tract.

Allergy is a state of altered reactivity in the host that results from interactions between an antigen and antibody.[59] Antigens stimulate the production of antibodies by penetrating the mucous membrane of either respiratory or gastrointestinal tracts. An antigen must be soluble in water and immunoglobulin E (IgE) is the antibody associated with allergy. When the IgE molecules on the surface of mast-cells recognise the antigen, calcium channels in the mast-cell membrane are opened and histamine is released. The arrival of neutrophils signals the inflammatory response that develops four hours later. These separate events explain the timing of both the immediate acute and the late asthmatic responses. Continued exposure to antigens like ragwood or grass pollens causes symptoms to persist.

Hay fever triggered by high pollen counts causes discomfort to a sizeable amount of people. Administration of antihistamines helps to alleviate the symptoms in many cases. Without such prophylactic measures, afflicted individuals can expect to have their competitive performance impaired by allergic reactions.

OVERVIEW

The precise effects of the many air pollutants on the many aspects of human performance, especially in elite athletes, have still not been adequately explored. Many of the studies reported have suffered from poor experimental design or illustrate the limitations of field work. In many cases the observations of concomitant changes in air concentrations, physiological responses and performance measures may have been coincidental rather than causal. Fitting them into a coherent pattern and relating this pattern to current environmental pollution data is a challenge for contemporary research groups.

Nevertheless, it is clear that the quality of the air breathed in can have an impact on exercise performance. Adverse environments may be encountered indoors as well as outdoors. There may also be consequences for human health: besides the pollutants discussed in this chapter, bacterial and viral infections can be transmitted through inspired air. At an extreme level, environmental pollution can be fatal. Many of the air pollutants related to industrial processes have been reduced since becoming subject to health and safety regulations. Others persist due to combinations of factors including climate, topography and human habitation. As well as natural defences against the adverse effects of air pollutants, artificial protective measures have also been adopted. These range from the imposition of environmental standards to the wearing of protective devices and ultimately to avoiding exposure altogether. Whilst individuals may have a tolerance to moderate concentrations of air pollutants, the extent to which humans have a capability to adapt to chronic exposure is not fully resolved.

References

1. Folinsbee LJ, Horvath SM, Raven PB et al. Influence of exercise and heat stress on pulmonary function during ozone exposure. J Appl Physiol (Respiration, Environmental Exerc Physiol) 1977; 43:409-413
2. Folinsbee LJ, Schelegle ES. Air pollutants and endurance performance. In: Shephard RJ, Astrand PO (eds). Endurance in sport. 2nd ed. Oxford: Blackwell, 2000:628-638
3. Sheppard D, Epstein J, Bethel RA et al. Tolerance to sulfur dioxide-induced broncho-constriction in subjects with asthma. Env Res 1983; 30:412-419
4. Sheppard D, Nadel JA, Boushey HA. Inhibition of sulfur dioxide – induced broncho-constriction by disodium cromoglycate in asthmatic subjects. Am Rev Resp Dis 1981; 12:257-259
5. Bedi JF, Horvath SM, Folinsbee LJ. Human exposure to sulfur dioxide and ozone: absence of synergistic effect. Arch Env Health 1982; 34:233-239
6. Koike A, Wasserman K, Armon Y et al. The work rate-dependent effect of carbon monoxide on ventilatory control during exercise. Respirat Physiol 1991; 85:169-183
7. Honigman B, Cromer R, Kurt TL. Carbon monoxide levels in athletes during exercise in an urban environment. J Air Pollution Control Assoc 1982; 32:77-79
8. Anderson E, Andelman R, Strauch J et al. Effect of low level carbon monoxide exposure on onset and duration of angina pectoris: a study of ten patients with ischaemic heart disease. Ann Intern Medicine 1973; 79:46-50
9. Nicholson JP, Case DB. Carboxyhaemoglobin levels in New York city runners. Physician Sportsmed 1983; 11:135-138
10. Waldman M, Weiss S, Articola W. A study of the health effects of bicycling in an urban atmosphere. US Department of Transport Report. Springfield: National Technical Information Service, 1977
11. Atkinson G. Air pollution and exercise. Sports Exerc Injury 1997; 3:2-8
12. Gill RMF. Carbon monoxide hazard in sub-Antarctic exploration. J Wilderness Med 1994; 5:4-10
13. Pugh LGCE. Carbon monoxide hazard in Antarctica. BMJ 1959; 1:192-196
14. Aranow W, Goldsmith J, Kern J et al. Effect of freeway travel on angina pectoris. Ann Intern Med 1972; 77:669-676
15. McCafferty WB. Air pollution and athletic performance. Springfield: Charles C Thomas, 1981
16. Atkinson G, Tindall N. Effects of cigarette smoke and transdermal nicotine absorption on the physiological responses to exercise. J Sports Sci 1997; 5:36-37
17. Goldsmith J, Cohen S. Epidemiological bases for possible air quality criteria for carbon monoxide. J Air Pollution Control Assoc, 1969; 19:704-713
18. Hazucha M, Folinsbee L, Seal E et al. Lung function and response of healthy women after sequential exposures to NO_2 and O_3. Am J Respir Crit Care Med 1994; 50:642-647
19. Lee K, Yanagisawa Y, Spengler J et al. Carbon monoxide and nitrogen dioxide exposures in indoor ice skating rinks. J Sports Sci 1994; 12:279-283

20. Persinger R, Blay W, Heintz N et al. Nitrogen dioxide induces death in lung epithelial cells in a density-dependent manner. Am J Resp Cell Mol Biol 2001, 24:583-590

21. Hedberg K, Hedberg C, Iber C et al. An outbreak of nitrogen dioxide-induced respiratory illness among ice hockey players. J Amer Med Assoc 1989; 262:3014-3017

22. Dewailly E, Allaire S, Nantel A. Nitrogen dioxide poisoning at a skating rink – Quebec. Canada CommunicableDiseases Report 1988; 14, 61-62

23. Egan E, Reilly T, Whyte G et al. Disorders of the menstrual cycle in elite female ice hockey players and skaters. Biol Rhythm Res 2003:34, 251-264

24. Brauer M, Spengler JD. Nitrogen dioxide exposures inside ice skating rinks. Am J Public Health 1994; 84:429-433

25. Atkinson G, MacLaren D, Taylor C. Blood lead levels of British competitive cyclists. Ergonomics 1994; 37:43-48

26. van Rensburg JP, van der Walt WH, van der Linde A et al. Lead absorption in distance runners exposed to motor vehicle exhaust fumes. S Afr J Res Sport Phys Ed Recr 1982; 5:21-44

27. Grobler SR, Maresky LS, Rossouw RJ. Blood lead levels of South African long-distance road runners. Arch Environ Health 1986; 41:155-158

28. Grant-White H. 'Joggitis', 'marathonitis' and marathon mania. S Afr Med J 1981; 59:849-850

29. Grobler SR, Maresky LS, Kotze TJ. Lead reduction of petrol and blood lead concentrations of athletes. Arch Environ Health 1992; 47:139-142

30. Stromme SB, Bredali K, Hawg H et al. Abnormally elevated blood lead level in competitive marksmen – a health hazard. Houston: Proceedings of the First World Olympic Congress in Sport Science, 1989:215-216

31. Georghiou PE, Blagden PA, Snow DA et al. Air levels and mutagenicity of PM-10 in an indoor ice arena. J Air Pollution Control Assoc 1989; 39:1583-1585

32. Afgado A, Bargada S, Romero PV et al. Exercise-induced airways narrowing and exposure to environmental tobacco smoke in school children. Amer J Epidemiol 1994; 140:409-417

33. MacNee W, Donaldson K. Particulate air pollution: injurious and protective mechanisms in the lung. In: Air pollution and health. Holgate T, Samet J, Koren H et al (eds). London: Academic Press, 1999:635-672

34. Bennet G. Oxygen contamination of high altitude aircraft cabins. Aerospace Med 1962; 33:969-973

35. Grievink L, Zijlstra A, Xiaodong K et al. Double-blind intervention trial on modulation of ozone effects on pulmonary function by antioxidant supplements. Amer J Epidemiol 1999; 149:306-314

37. Hackney JD, Linn WS, Buckley RD et al. Studies in adaptation to ambient oxidant air pollution effects of ozone exposure in Los Angeles resident vs new arrivals. Environ Health Perspect 1976; 18:141-146

38. Hackney JD, Linn WS, Karuza SK et al. Effects of ozone exposure in Canadians and Southern Californians: evidence for adaptation? Arch Environ Health 1977; 32:110-116

39. Folinsbee LJ, Raven PB. Exercise and air pollution. J Sports sci 1984;2:57-75

40 Moussiopoulos N, Papagrigoriou S. Urban air pollution: Athens 2004 air quality. California: EnviroComp Institute, 2002

41. Haymes EM, Wells C. Environment and human performance. Champaign, Illinois: Human Kinetics, 1986

42. Raven PB, Gliner JA, Sutton JC. Dynamic lung function changes following long-term work in polluted environments. Environ Res 1976; 12:18-25

43. Reilly T, Atkinson G, Waterhouse J. Biological rhythms and exercise. Oxford: Oxford University Press, 1997

44. Muns G, Singer P, Wolf F et al. Impaired nasal mucociliary clearance in long-distance runners. Int J Sports Med 1995; 16:209-213

45. Landrigan PJ, McKinney AS, Hopkins LC. Chronic lead absorption: result of poor ventilation in an indoor pistol range. J Amer Med Assoc 1975; 234:394-397

46. Brauer M, Spengler JD, Lee K et al. Air pollutant exposures inside ice hockey rinks: exposure assessment and reduction strategies. In: Safety in ice hockey. 2nd vol. Casteldi CR, Bishop PJ, Hoerner EF (eds). Philadelphia: ASTM, 1993:142-158

47. Samet J, Hatch G, Horstman D et al. Effect of antioxidant supplementation on ozone-induced lung injury in human subjects. Amer J Resp Critical Care Med 2001; 164:819-825

48. Hawkins LH, Barker T. Air ions and human performance. Ergonomics 1978; 21:273-278

49. Sovijarvi ARA, Rossel S, Hyvarin J et al. Effect of air ionization on heart rate and perceived exertion during a bicycle exercise test: a double blind cross-over study. Europ J Appl Physiol 1979; 41:285-291

50. Inbar O, Roistein A, Dlin R et al. The effects of negative air ions on various physiological functions during work in hot environments. Int J Biometeorol 1982; 26:153-156

51. Krueger AP, Reed EJ. Biological impact of small air ions. Science 1976; 193:1209-1213

52. Strydom NB, Kotze HF, Vanderwall WH et al. Effects of ascorbic acid on rate of heat acclimatisation. J Appl Physiol 1976; 41:202-205

53. Krueger AP, Smith RF. Negative air ion effects on the concentration and metabolism of 5-hydroxytryptamine in the mammalian respiratory tract. J Gen Physiol 1960; 44:269-276

54. Reilly T, Stevenson C. An investigation of the effects of negative air ions on responses to submaximal exercise at different times of day. J Hum Ergol 1993; 22:1-9

55. Charry JM. Biological effects of small air ions – a review of findings and methods. Environ Res 1984; 34:351-389

56. Reilly T, Brooks GA. Exercise and circadian variation in body temperature measures. Int J Sports Med 1986; 7:358-362

57. Reilly T, Brooks GA. Investigation of circadian rhythms in metabolic responses to exercise. Ergonomics 1982; 25:1093-1107

58. Yates CA, Herbert J. Differential circadian rhythms in pineal hypothalamic 5HT induced by artificial photoperiods or melatonin. Nature 1966; 262:219-220

59. Harries M. The lung in sport. In: Oxford textbook of sports medicine. 2nd ed. Harries M, Williams C, Stanish WD et al (eds). Oxford: Oxford University Press, 1998:321-326

Chapter 9

Noise

CHAPTER CONTENTS

Introduction 165
The physics of noise 166
The anatomy of the ear 167
Hearing tests 169
Types of deafness 170
The ergonomics context 172

Sports or recreational activities
   involving noise hazards 173
Protection and noise control 176
Overview 178

INTRODUCTION

The concept of noise as an environmental pollutant is relatively new. Sources include machinery, jet engines, motor vehicles, subways, radios and sirens. There are also natural sources of loud noise such as thunderclaps and in a sports context, the vocal responses of spectators to game events. In motor sports and rallies, noise is an inevitable corollary of the events themselves.

Noise may be defined as unwanted sound. In this respect the concept covers both noise as an environmental stressor and as interference with oral communication. Its meaning in communication theory is that noise is considered as 'that auditory stimulus' bearing no information relationship to the presence or completion of the immediate task. This concept applies equally to task-related sounds that contain no relevant information and to sounds that are not task-related. In designing communication systems, engineers endeavour to minimize noise within the communication channel and to maximize the signal-to-noise ratio. The concept of signal-to-noise ratio has been used in this generic sense in both the biological and behavioural sciences.

It is mainly in its sense of physical sound that we understand noise. Noise can be the cause of acute adverse effects on (temporary threshold shifts in) hearing, or of more serious long-term hearing damage. As a chronic irritant it may have adverse effects on health, and cause disturbance of sleep. It is therefore important that methods of dealing with noise, whether at source or subsequent attenuation, are addressed. The paradox is that sound can also have tremendously positive effects, whether by emotive means such as cheering one's sports team or experiencing the pleasurable sensations of one's favourite music. Its subjective effects may be combined, for example when loud music is played on public address systems to direct the mood of the spectators prior to or during sports competitions.

There is often an emotional or aesthetic component to the sounds experienced in certain sports. This response may be reflected in the thud of an arrow hitting its target dead centre or a sweetly hit golf shot, resounding with the sharp impact loading of the ball being hit by the face of the club. Indeed, Shannon and Axe[1] claimed that a simple acoustic drop test offers a convenient method of determining the elastic properties of golf balls and their cores. Similarly, the sound of a ball on a bat made of willow has special connotations for followers of cricket.

In this chapter, the structure of sound is first explained before the mechanisms for translating sound characteristics into meaningful human communication are explained. Sport as a source of noise and risk to hearing is considered and various means of protecting against noise are described.

THE PHYSICS OF NOISE

Sound consists of pressure waves originating from a vibrating object. These waves travel through an elastic medium at about 760 mph (338 m/s) as a succession of waves of compression and expansion, and are transmitted into the ear where they generate nerve signals that are perceived as sound. Pure tones are sine waves, defined in terms of amplitude and frequency. Complex tones are made up of superimposed sine waves.

The displacement of the molecules of the transmitting medium from their place of rest determines the amplitude of vibration of a sound wave. The energy involved in that displacement in turn determines the intensity of the sound. Subjective sensation is equated with loudness; the greater the amplitude, the greater the sound pressure level. Sound pressure is expressed in dynes/cm whereas sound is measured in decibels (dB) or 0.1 bel. Frequency is indicated in hertz (Hz), representing the number of waves arriving each second. The subjective sensation of frequency is indicated by pitch. Sound is generated by vibrations from some source and transmitted through the atmosphere to the ear. For frequencies of 20-15000 Hz, sound is heard by the human ear. Intelligible speech lies within the bandwidth of 620-4800 Hz, but the main frequencies used in speech fall in range of 300 to 3500 Hz. Ultrasound indicates mechanical vibration in excess of 20,000 beats.

On the decibel scale, arbitrary zero is the faintest sound that can be heard by the human ear at 1000 Hz; this value represents 0.00002 Newtons/m^2 (0.0002 dynes/cm^2). The smallest change appreciated by the ear is about 1 dB, whether the change is in faint or loud sound. The decibel is a physical measure of sound intensity on a logarithmic pressure ratio scale. The scale and its zero point are chosen to correspond to subjective phenomena, although the scale is physical in nature and based on amplitude.

Table 9.1 Decibel ratings of sounds

Sound	Rating (decibels)
Absolute silence	0
Watch ticking	20
Residential street, no traffic	40
Stream	50
Automobile at 10 m	60
Conversation at 1 m	70
Loud radio	80
Truck at 5 m	90
Car horn at 5 m	100
Pneumatic hammer at 1 m	120
Amplified rock music	130
Propeller airplane at 5 m	130
Jet aircraft at takeoff	150+

The loudest sound is one million million times the intensity of the faintest we can hear. The decibel scale takes this into account and is logarithmic (Table 9.1). Therefore, tenfold increases, from 1 to 10, from 10 to 100, and from 100 to 1000, are represented by changes of 10 dB. Doubling the intensity corresponds to about 3 dB. A 20-fold change = 10 + 3 = 13 dB; whereas a 200-fold change = 20 + 3 = 23 dB. Listening becomes uncomfortable at 120 dB.

Loudness is measured in phons. The phon scale takes account of variations in frequency as well as amplitude and is identical to the dB scale only for tones of 1000 Hz. It is not linear in subjective terms (40 phons is not twice as loud as 20). The phon scale was developed by Fletcher and Munson[2] as equal loudness contours. They obtained judgement of subjects with regard to sounds of different frequencies and intensities deemed to have equal loudness.

THE ANATOMY OF THE EAR

The ear's function is to convert the pressure waves of sound into neural signals for transmission to the brain. The auditory system converts pressure changes in the air, via pressure changes in a liquid medium, into pulses which

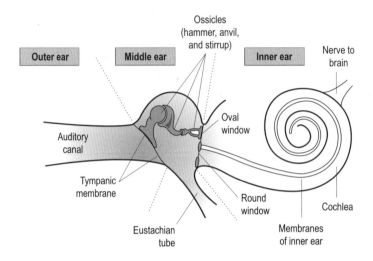

Figure 9.1 Schematic drawing of the ear showing auditory canal through which sound waves travel to tympanic membrane, which in turn vibrates the ossicles of the middle ear. This vibration is transmitted through the membrane of the oval window to the cochlea, where the vibrations are transmitted by liquid through membranes to sensitive hair cells, which send nerve impulses to the brain.

contain pitch and loudness information. This feat is accomplished by a series of transformations:

- into mechanical movement;
- into hydrostatic pressure;
- into an electrical signal or neural signal.

Transformations occur in the outer, middle and inner ear. The *outer ear* consists of the pinna (external ear) which is a tube connecting to the interior of the head. The tympanic membrane or eardrum closes the tube at its inner end. The pinna collects sound waves and passes them through the narrow canal to the ear drum. The membrane vibrates when small sound waves fall on it. Vibrations are transmitted to the *middle ear* – an air-filled cavity that is separated from the outer ear by the eardrum and opens to the throat. To its centre is attached the malleus, one of three small bones – the malleus (hammer), incus (anvil) and stapes (stirrup). These bones make up a mechanical linear linkage which transmits movement from the eardrum to the oval window on the other side. It is important for the functioning of the oval window that the mid-ear pressure equals that of the environment, so the middle ear is connected to the back of the throat by the Eustachian tube which is opened by the act of swallowing.

The *inner ear* is a small, snail-shaped organ filled with fluid containing a membrane on which about 2500 specialized cells are located. The most important part is the cochlea, a coiled whorl-like structure similar to a snail's shell. There are $2^1/2$ turns tapering towards its end. The wide end of the cochlea abuts the middle ear, at the so-called oval and round windows, which are apertures covered by a membrane (see Figure 9.1). The spaces within the cochlea are filled with two types of fluid, known as perilymph and endolymph, respectively. The former closely resembles cerebrospinal fluid whilst endolymph, possessing a high concentration of potassium and a low concentration of sodium, is more like intracellular fluid. The cochlea has two membranes, the tectorial (upper) and basilar (lower). These membranes form the Organ of Corti which runs the length of the cochlea. The basilar membrane is narrowest and stiffest close to the oval window but broadens and becomes more flexible as it extends through the cochlea. The basilar membrane will pulse at a specific point along its length according to the frequency of the input at the oval window. The basilar membrane vibrates from changes in hydrostatic pressure in the fluid. Hair cells or cilia above the basilar membrane are embedded in an inner single row and an outer three rows. As the basilar membrane pulses, the cilia are pushed up against the tectorial membrane and bent over in the process, which triggers the propagation of a nerve impulse from the hair cell. Individual hair cells attached to ganglia then propagate neural transmission from the cochlea via the auditory nerve. The signal is transmitted to the auditory cortex located in the temporal lobe of the brain.

Sounds pass from outer ear into middle ear and on to inner ear in 0.001 s. The middle ear has a natural reflex to protect against sudden loud noises. The tensor tympani and stapedius muscles act to hold the connections of the ossicles rigid and the eardrum stiff in order to reduce the propagation of loud sound waves into the cochlea. These muscles are attached respectively to the malleus and stapes. When these muscles are stimulated to contract, they damp movements of the ossicular chain and so decrease the sensitivity of the hearing apparatus. This action protects the ear against damage, except in cases of sudden unexpected loud noise. Their response time is of the order of 100 ms, so some damage to sensitive aural structures may occur before the auditory attenuating reflex can become active.

HEARING TESTS

There are two basic methods of measuring hearing.

Simple hearing tests

Voice and whisper test The experimenter speaks or whispers to the subject at different voice intensities and at different distances. The experimenter is out of sight and the subject is asked to repeat what was said.

Watch-tick test, coin-click test and others Such tests may serve for purposes of rough assessment but lack standardization. More objective tests are usually required.

Clinical tests Two types of test are used to differentiate conduction loss and sensorineural loss. They entail recording responses to a vibrating tuning fork placed against the middle of the forehead or against the mastoid process. The subject is asked either to localize the sound to one ear or indicate when the sound dies out.

Audiometer tests

An audiometer This is an instrument to measure hearing at various frequencies. It reproduces, through earphones, pure tones of different frequencies and intensities. As intensity is increased or decreased, the subject is asked to indicate when he/she can hear the tone or when it ceases to be audible. It is then possible to determine, for each frequency tested, the lowest intensity that can just barely be heard i.e. the threshold for the frequency.

Speech audiometry Direct or recorded speech is reproduced to earphones or a loudspeaker and the intensity controlled. Various types of speech intelligibility tests are then performed. An intelligibility index concludes the percentage of spoken material that can be understood. The following should be noted when audiometry tests are employed to survey noise conditions:

- It is essential that there should be a noise-free interval from the last exposure (24-36 hours) to separate temporary from permanent threshold shifts. A temporary threshold shift is a transient loss of hearing which returns to normal after 36 hours.
- There can be large differences of hearing loss in individuals exposed to the same noise stimulus for the same noise exposure time. No test exists to predict those who will be particularly susceptible.
- Individuals showing ear disease should be excluded from surveys of noisy conditions as these could confound the measurements.

TYPES OF DEAFNESS

Middle ear deafness is a moderate deafness. Its cause is usually stiffening or damping of the ossicles. There may be an infection in the middle ear, Eustachian tube obstruction, or perforation of the ear drum. The increased resistance that ensues impairs low tones rather than high tones. Provided the inner ear is intact and functions normally, medical treatment with antibiotics or surgical repair of the drum will return hearing to normal. Also, use of amplification by means of a hearing aid will be successful.

Nerve deafness may affect the perception of all sounds or only a range of the spectrum. Damage is either to special receptor cells or to the nerve trunks supplying input to the brain's hearing centre. Causes of inner ear cell damage may include infections such as measles and mumps. Certain medicaments (streptomycin, enomycia, quinine, salicylates) may also be implicated. Head injuries, especially skull fractures, can also be a cause of destruction of nerves.

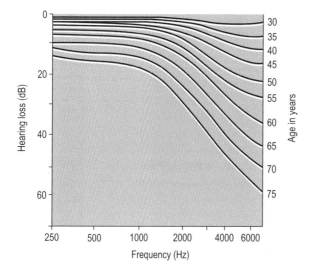

Figure 9.2 The amount of hearing loss due to presbycousis with increasing age. After Oborne DJ. Ergonomics at work[4]

Exposure to high noise levels is particularly destructive to the receptor cells in the inner ear.

Exposure to high noise levels leads to a temporary threshold shift. If the loss continues, it becomes a permanent threshold shift. A rise in the hearing threshold takes place 0.15 octaves higher than the noise tone. In nerve deafness of this kind, hearing loss occurs first in high tones over about 4000 Hz which, as this is above speech frequencies, passes unnoticed. If the repetition rate of impact noise is longer than 0.1 s, the middle ear muscles will have time to contract and protect the ear. They will not have time to do so if the noise is unexpected.

The duration of the sound pressure wave is the key separating steady state from impulse noise. In firearm discharge, the intensity of noise peaks within 0.2 to 2 ms. The time required for the middle ear muscles to contract and dampen the mobility of the tympanic membrane and attached ossicles is 100-150 ms. Clearly this is not possible in the case of gunfire.

Dullness of hearing may be associated with a ringing or buzzing sensation. Once the receptor cells have degenerated, no recovery of hearing is possible. The cells affected no longer generate electrical impulses and so no signals are transmitted to the hearing centre. Amplification devices then provide no alleviation.

Presbyacousis refers to a loss of hearing due to age. There is increasing deterioration at the higher frequencies (4000 Hz or above) and losses do not interfere with speech communication until about age 65 years or so. The normal human speech range spans 300-3500 Hz[3] but speech for both males

> **Box 9.1 A list of factors which can cause annoyance either in combination or singly**
>
> Loudness
>
> High pitch
>
> Harshness (lack of musical quality)
>
> Discrete tones in broadband noise
>
> Irregularity of loudness, pitch, rhythm
>
> Frequent repetition
>
> Abruptness of starting or ending
>
> Unexpectedness
>
> Uncertainty about source
>
> Inappropriate time of day/night
>
> Disturbance of activity (e.g. speech/sleep)
>
> Susceptibility of hearer (e.g. during illness)
>
> Emotional implications (e.g. fear of crash)
>
> Noise being unnecessary, avoidable, deliberate or too long

and females tends to predominate at about 500 Hz[4] (see Figure 9.2). Cutting off the top of the speech frequencies (1000-3000 Hz) results in whispers being inaudible and difficulty in word discrimination – especially 's', 'f', 'm' and 'th' sounds. Loss of hearing due to age is additive to that produced by loud noise.

THE ERGONOMICS CONTEXT

Noise in industrial or leisure contexts is important for the following reasons.

People do not like it – it causes annoyance (see Box 9.1). It may then be related to the morale of the workforce or to the enjoyment of exercise.

Annoyance is caused by loudness, high pitch, discrete tones in broadband noise, irregularity, abruptness at the start or end of sound, unexpectedness, disturbance of concentration (such as while waiting for a sprint start or taking a penalty kick), emotional implications (hearing the noise of a crash), and unnecessary or prolonged noise.

Community noise such as traffic or aircraft noise, for example near airports, is a particular nuisance. On the whole, the louder the noise, the more people complain. Nevertheless there are large differences between individuals in what they find annoying. Most people find high-pitched noises more annoying than low-pitched, and intermittent and sudden noise more annoying than steady, prolonged noise. Also, sounds from unknown sources or due to thoughtlessness are especially distracting.

It damages hearing – although people may fail to notice the damage for various reasons. Firstly, it develops slowly, except for when an eardrum is ruptured by violent sound. Secondly, it may be limited to faint sounds. Thirdly, the effect may not be the same for all frequencies.

It has other health implications – health may also be impaired due to repeated or chronic exposure to noise. Impulsive noise can cause increased blood pressure or damage to blood vessels. Stress hormones are also elevated when noise is persistent. A long-term effect of noise may be disrupted sleep and a deterioration in general health.

People may work less well – although research results are contradictory. The main adverse effect in industrial tasks is on accuracy rather than on speed. The maximum noise level recommended for an office environment is 60 dB. At 90 dB, conversation becomes difficult and verbal instructions may be misunderstood. Another effect is that sounds that most frequently occur cause distraction and disturbance of oral communication. In cybernetic terms, unwanted sounds are considered as distracting or interfering with communication, altering the signal-to-noise ratio is by attenuating the signal and amplifying the noise.

SPORTS OR RECREATIONAL ACTIVITIES INVOLVING NOISE HAZARDS

Listening to loud music

Whether music is perceived as too loud will depend, to a large extent, on age and taste. Discotheques have been criticized for highly amplified music. Limited evidence suggests that discos, clubs and pop concerts may involve a small but definite hearing risk. At discos, peak noise levels of 120 dB are not unknown and average levels for a session often exceed 105 dB. Using data prepared for industrial noise exposure, a person who spends 15 min/day subjected to continuous noise of 105 dB runs the same risk of hearing damage as one spending 8 hours at 90 dB. Young people may only go 'clubbing' or to discotheques once or twice a week, so their hearing is rested in the meantime. Individuals who are subjected to high noise levels during the day and add to this disco or 'clubbing' noise in the evening are at greater risk. Noise levels are also a concern for workers in nightclubs (disc jockeys and audio-visual technicians) who may get little respite from high noise doses during the conduct of their occupations and regularly experience tinnitus, a lingering, ringing sensation in the ears.

Safety measures recommended for those attending clubs, discotheques or pop concerts include avoiding standing close to loudspeakers, and resting the ears occasionally by adjourning to a quiet room or to a distance from outdoor loudspeakers. This advice applies particularly if buzzing in the ears is experienced.

Shooting

The risk of hearing damage is recognized by governing bodies, who advise participants to use ear protection. A 0.22 rifle (one of the less noisy weapons in sporting use) can produce peak sound pressure levels of 130-140 dB. Pistols and rifles of larger calibre produce noise in the 140-160 dB range. Despite the short duration, these represent high values of impulsive sound and significant noise levels. There is evidence that shooting regularly with a 12-bore shotgun damages the ears of recreational participants. The only way of avoiding risk is to wear ear protectors.

The head provides some degree of protection for the averted ear in rifle shooting. Turning the head, as done when firing a shoulder-held weapon, provides a 'head-shadow' for one of the ears.[5] This shadow can produce attenuations of 25-30 dB at frequencies above 1000 Hz but is negligible below this frequency. In contrast, a pistol shooter keeps the head squarely facing the target, placing both ears equally at risk.

Motor racing

Race-track meetings, hill climbs, motorcross, grass-track racing and other racing events not held on public roads are invariably noisy. Without the shriek of engines or tyres, these sports might not be as attractive to spectators. Noise levels reach values above 100 dB. The duration of exposure may be relatively short for spectators. The people most at risk are drivers, mechanics and track officials, though spectators also may receive high doses if positioned near the track. Mechanics and officials should wear ear-protectors, like those developed for noisy industrial situations. A sensible ploy would be for competitors to wear safety helmets; earplugs of the glass-down variety are suitable.

Motor cycling

Motor cyclists are exposed to noise levels well in excess of the 85 dB permitted for an eight-hour working day under the Health and Safety at Work Act of 1989. Noise from the machinery is satisfactorily controlled by the Auto-cycle Union and the main hazard is associated with turbulent airflow around the rider's helmet. This low-frequency 'wind noise' amounts to 90 dB at 56 km/h.[6]

Hearing loss induced by exposure to noise of such intensity is first evident as a drop in the audiogram between the frequencies of 3000 and 6000 Hz. The loss of hearing spreads to frequencies on either side of this region as the damage progresses. McCombe and Binnington[6] showed that grand prix motorcyclists (20 out of 44 examined) had hearing losses greater than expected for age-matched controls. The hearing deficit tended to increase with racing experience. Less than 40% of the riders were regular users of earplugs. Many riders choosing not to use earplugs expressed concern about their effects on perceptions of other environmental sounds, in particular the engine and exhaust of the motorcycles. This concern was not corroborated by the views of those using hearing protection.

'Do-it-yourself' activities

There is an increasing use of power tools for carrying out 'do-it-yourself' jobs more quickly and with less effort. Some of the tools are noisy and if used for lengthy periods can be hazardous. Ear protectors are recommended by the Noise Advisory Council. Noisy machines include some motor mowers, chainsaws, electric hedge trimmers, circular saws, sanding machines (especially when used on metal surfaces), hammers (in certain circumstances) and percussion tools. Used outdoors, the only person at risk is the operator. Ear protection is essential with chain saws. Risks are greater when power equipment is used indoors – in workshops and garages with little sound-absorbing material. For the average handyman or handywoman, it is recommended to use machines for short periods of time only.

Swimming in indoor pools

People who frequently visit public baths which have inadequate acoustical treatment may be vulnerable to noise pollution. Sound levels during busy periods may be very high. Peak levels of noise in such baths may be 100 dB but 90-92 dB levels are common. Sensible precautions are to avoid lengthy stays during busy periods, and to wear rubber ear protectors of the kind designed to keep out water. These protective devices must be a tight fit to be effective.

Snowmobiling

Snowmobiles represent a convenient form of transport over terrain covered in snow. These vehicles are used by mountain rangers for transportation and also by competitors in snowmobile racing. Snowmobiles may produce up to 136 dB at full throttle (26 horse-power engine). Temporary threshold shifts (TTS) lasting 4-14 days are found in racing drivers. A range of 0-20 dB TTS was found at about 2000 and 4000 Hz. This applied to both drivers and riders.[7] Levels of sound pressure exceeded by 10 dB the Damage Risk Conditions of the American Committee of Hearing and Bioacoustics for the Speech Frequency Range (500-2000 Hz). Data suggest drivers should not exceed 11 minutes of snowmobiling at a time.

Unrestrained snowmobile operation would represent a significant noise dosage for those exposed. Such a hazard is additional to the risk of animal and human deaths, not to mention the ecological damage due to these machines.

Exercise and music

Music can influence the mood of spectators at sports events. This possible effect is exemplified by the use of loud popular music as a means of arousing the audience prior to the start of competitions. Careful selection of particular songs or tunes can also underline an individual athlete's achievements, for example the 200 m victory of Michael Johnson at the Atlanta Olympics in 1996 where the warm-down of the gold medallist was accompanied by the amplified chorus of 'You're Unbelievable'. Spectators at World Cup soccer tournaments anticipate the rhythmic sound of samba music to accompany the performance of the Brazilian national team. Such musical evocations add to the excitement and atmosphere of the games.

Background music is used in leisure environments to 'soften the atmosphere' and create a feeling of relaxation. Music is also used by professional football teams in the dressing rooms before a match to help the players' mental preparation for the forthcoming game. The difficulty presented here is a need for an appropriate choice of music that has a positive effect on all individuals. This problem is avoided when individuals use their own headphones and select their preferred style of music to suit the desired mood.

Music may also influence the individual performer's response to exercise. Besides increasing arousal in a competitive context, it may be a distracting influence on strenuous training, dissociating one's perceptions to external rather than internal stimuli associated with perceived exertion. Alternatively, under light to moderate exercise intensities as in walking or jogging, listening to music through headphones can have a relaxing effect and assist compliance to the exercise programme. The impact of music on the performer seems to depend on its type and the performance context.

Slow, soft music tends to decrease physiological responses to sub-maximal exercise, particularly evident in a lowered heart rate. Further, exercise to exhaustion has been increased when accompanied by soft, slow music compared to fast, loud music or to a control condition.[8] Fast rock music tends to elevate heart rate responses to submaximal exercise.[9] Whilst soft, slow music has a favourable effect on perceived exertion during exercise of light intensity, the influence of accompanying music tends to disappear when maximal exercise is undertaken.

PROTECTION AND NOISE CONTROL

The appropriate means of engineering protection are controlling the source of noise or isolating it. The individual may be protected by use of ear devices.

Control at source

Proper design of equipment, regular maintenance, attention to lubrication and use of rubber mountings are helpful in controlling noise at source. Hard walls, floors and ceilings reflect sound and increase noise and should be addressed at the design stage. These problems can also be treated by creating sound traps, especially by means of a rough, porous surface. Use of thick carpets and padded furniture can be helpful.

Isolation of noise

Noise may be isolated by acoustical treatment of the environment, use of sound absorbers and proper layout of equipment. These remedies are employed to correct for errors of omission at the design stage.

Ear protection

Effectiveness of ear protection is limited to 35 dB at 250 Hz and 60 dB at higher frequencies. A wide range of safety devices is available.

Earplugs (prefabricated) These are available in a variety of sizes, made of soft, flexible material. The plugs must provide a snug, airtight and comfortable fit. They should be non-toxic and have a smooth surface for cleaning. The V51R (soft plastic) model is available in five sizes. Noise reduction depends on fit and can vary by 10 dB. The plug may be sited accurately by putting it into the external ear, which opens and straightens the ear canal.

Malleable and disposable ear plugs Glass-wool, wax, cotton or a mixture of these is used to form a small cone by hand and the apex is then inserted into the middle ear. This type of plug is capable of providing similar reduction as the pre-fabricated type if made and sited correctly. Glass-wool or 'glass-down' is the best type. Glass-down is a form of glass-wool in which fibres are so fine they form a material of down-like softness reported to be harmless to the delicate skin of the middle ear. Glass-wool is not recommended in areas having high intermittent noise levels or where it is necessary to remove and reinsert protective devices regularly during work periods. Cotton wool by itself provides little attenuation; if waxed it is a little better but still unsatisfactory.

Individually-moulded earplugs These are made of silicon rubber and are moulded in a permanent form within the ear canal so the plug conforms to the shape of the canal. If correctly made and sited, this device can be better than the prefabricated design. The degree of protection depends on expertise of moulding and usually five or six separate fitting attempts are required. The silicone rubber is supplied with a curing agent and the two are then mixed to a putty-like consistency before inserting into the ear. The 'cure' time is about ten minutes and no jaw movements are allowed during this period. On removal, the plug is in a permanent form. It is comfortable to wear.

Ear muffs Rigid cups which cover the external ear and are held against the head by a spring-loaded adjustable band. The seal to the head is made with soft cushions that envelop the whole ear. The fluid-seal type is best: this device is a plastic ring containing fluid such as glycerin, which fits around the ear and minimizes sound leakage. To overcome the high-frequency resonances within the cup, the enclosed volume is filled with absorbent material (plastic foam). The seal material must be non-irritant and non-toxic and unaffected by sweat. Ear muffs provide the greatest protection but the noise reduction of muffs is dependent, firstly, on the cup-head seal (this seal is reduced when muffs are worn over long hair or spectacle frames) and secondly, on the force with which the cups are pressed against the side of the head. The maximum noise reduction afforded by ear muffs is 35 dB at 240 Hz, 60 dB at higher frequencies. Ear muffs fit most people, are suitable for people frequently moving into and out of high noise levels and can be worn by people unable to wear ear plugs because of infection of the outer ear canal or meatus.

Helmets These prevent sounds reaching high levels due to conduction via skull bones.

The best protection is afforded by a combination of helmet and ear plugs. Kirk[10] monitored helmet-mounted ear muffs in loggers over a 12-month period and concluded that the devices could be safely used as an effective form of protecting against chainsaw noise.

OVERVIEW

Typical noise levels within the hearing range vary from explosions (about 160 dB) to a whisper at 1 m (20 dB). Noise in excess of 85 to 90 dB is a potential threat to hearing. Noise may be annoying and hence hinder performance or interfere with communication and thereby impair safety at much lower levels. The nature and context of noise, more than its intensity, will affect how the individual perceives it. Normally, noise will be distracting when the individual is attempting to focus on a particular task or activity. Conversely, noise may partly counter the effects of sleep deprivation and keep the individual awake. Generally, certain high frequencies are more stressful than low-frequency noise of a similar intensity. Noise in sport can either distract the performer (for example, crowd noise may precipitate a false start in a sprinter poised on the starting blocks waiting for the starter's gun to fire) or motivate an entire team. The phenomenon of home advantage, whereby the team benefits from playing at its local competitive venue, may be explained in part by the vocal support from home supporters. There is evidence that the noise generated by a partisan crowd can also influence the decisions of football referees.[11] When noise endangers the health or hearing of the athlete or recreation participant, it cannot be accepted, and protective measures should be employed. Furthermore, attention to acoustical features can bring appreciable benefits to the design of indoor sports arenas and to conference rooms.

References

1. Shannon K, Axe JD. On the acoustic signature of golf ball impact. J Sports Sci 2002; 20:629-633
2. Fletcher H, Munson WA. Loudness, its definition, measurement and calculation. J Acoustical Soc America 1933; 5:82-108
3. Berne RM, Levy MN, Koeppen BM et al. Physiology. 4th ed. St Louis: CV Mosby, 1998
4. Oborne DJ. Ergonomics at work. 3rd ed. Chichester: John Wiley, 1995
5. Keim RJ. Impulse noise and neurosensory hearing loss. Calif Med 1970; 113:16-19
6. McCombe AW, Binnington J. Hearing loss in Grand Prix motorcyclists: occupational hazard or sports injury? Brit J Sports Med 1994; 28:35-37
7. Rabideau CF. Human, machine and environmental aspects of snowmobile design and utilization. Hum Factors 1974; 16:481-494
8. Copeland BL, Franks BD. Effects of types and intensities of background music on treadmill endurance. J Sports Med Phys Fitn 1991; 31:100-103
9. Wilson C, Aiken LC. The effects of intensity levels upon physiological and subjective response to rock music. J Music Therapy 1977; t4:60-76
10. Kirk P. Earmuff effectiveness against chainsaw noise over a 12-month period. Appl Ergon 1993; 24:279-283
11. Nevill AM, Balmer NJ, Williams AM. Crowd influence on decisions in association football. Lancet 1999; 353:1416

Chapter 10

Living and exercising in hostile environments

CHAPTER CONTENTS

Introduction 181
A balance with nature? 183
Acclimatization and habituation 185
Analyzing lifestyle 186

Environmental stresses in combination 188
Conclusion 190

INTRODUCTION

In literature and religious writing there is an idyll where people are totally in tune with their enviroment. In fact, enviromental characteristics rarely feature in accounts of Shangri La, Caliban's Island or the Garden of Eden. Instead the emphasis is laid on the tranquil feelings of the individuals placed within the mythical environment and their temporary release from earthly cares. The tourist, too, is sometimes deluded into thinking that a 'heaven on Earth' has been found, whether this is in the remote areas of the Rockies, the waterfalls of Iceland (see Figure 10.1), a secluded Caribbean beach or the 'old town' of one of the old European cities. Whilst the reality is that this 'paradise' is illusory, people do generally feel at one with a particular place, whether by birth, settlement or immigration. In other words, there is 'no place like home'.

Apart from scenery and aesthetics, the major factor facilitating 'oneness' with the local environment is probably the weather. This is the reason why hordes of visitors are attracted towards sites where the scenery is pleasant and the climatic conditions are good. There is a particular attraction towards the seaside and to sunny locations in the summer. Venues that offer splendid scenery and opportunities for active recreation are also hugely attractive (see Figure 10.2). In winter, the alternative is an active holiday, walking in the hills or skiing on the mountain slopes. Yet these activities are not totally customer-friendly in that accidents are possible in the water, sunburn and skin cancer result from over-exposure to solar radiation, and physiological homeostasis is threatened if the traveller is unprepared for cold conditions in wilderness.

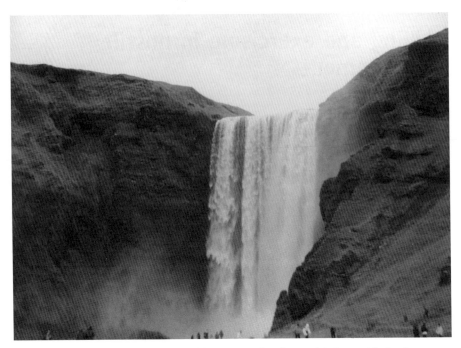

Figure 10.1 Its natural waterfalls provide an attraction for tourists in rural Iceland

There is a tendency in humans to become dissatisfied with stability and a reluctance to stay permanently in the relative comfort of the status quo. There seems to be an intrinsic existentialist drive to seek out new challenges and explore and even exceed one's apparent limits. This drive leads some explorers into the altitude of the high mountains, and others to the extreme cold and isolation of the polar regions or to the extreme heat of the desert.

All areas of the world have now been mapped, although there are places on it where few humans have ventured. Even the remote and uninviting areas provide challenges for those who are competitive and adventurous. The various forms of altitude records, underwater exploration and desert races are testimony to the quest to operate in extremes. The Marathon de Sable (over a distance of 240 km) is organized each year in the Sahara desert, and the Iditarod sled-races with huskies are held annually in Alaska. Adventure canoeing through river rapids can be exhilarating to watch and participate in, but calls for considerable expertise to be done safely.

Even major sports tournaments have been held under demanding environmental conditions. The summer Olympic Games have been held in conditions that pose problems of altitude, heat and pollution. Athletes must not only train for the physiological demands of the event but also prepare to cope with the expected climatic conditions. The environmental conditions have been isolated and dealt with separately within the previous chapters of this book. In this chapter, some attempt is made to integrate the environmental factors within a holistic perspective.

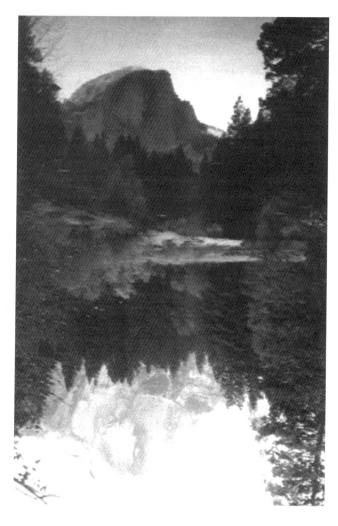

Figure 10.2 Yosemite Valley in the Sierras - a natural attraction for hikers, back-packers and rock climbers. Stunning natural scenery and seemingly incessant sunshine contribute to the magnetic attraction of California

A BALANCE WITH NATURE?

A concern among so-called environmentalists is the damage that visitors unwittingly cause on the terrain that initially attracted them. The wilderness may be spoiled by trekkers, either over-using the unrestricted tracks or leaving refuse behind them. Even so, there is a code of behaviour amongst dedicated ramblers and hill walkers to care for the countryside and not to degrade any of its beauties with unwanted clutter.

The many expeditions to climb the high mountains are other examples of how the wilderness can be spoiled. The hundreds of expeditions to the slopes of Mount Everest have marked their presence with little regard for ecology along the way. There are safety considerations too: for example, recreational participants who ski off-piste may unintentionally trigger an avalanche and put others at risk.

Human activities impinge on the overall environment in more subtle ways. Global climate change and the hole in the ozone layer have left individuals in the sun more exposed to the adverse effects of ultraviolet radiation. The loss of the ice-shelves in the polar regions has meant that explorers must now time their expeditions with ever more attention to seasonal changes. The record temperature of 37.9°C in London during August 2003 alerted the public to the phenomenon of global warming, global temperatures having risen by an average 0.5°C over the last 50 years. Most experts now believe that such weather patterns are caused by the build up in the atmosphere of carbon dioxide and other industrial gases. There is worldwide concern about the need to implement an international code of practice (the Kyoto Agreement) for controlling emissions of greenhouse gases, if long-term environmental disaster is to be avoided.

The planners of sports events may sometimes have to bow to the vagaries of the weather. Rain regularly stops play in outdoor lawn tennis and cricket matches. Lightning and thunderstorms halt events where it would be dangerous to continue, for example golfers sheltering under trees during an electrical storm. Storms cause havoc with sailing and yachting races, but in 'Round the World' races the competitors may be completely exposed. Current state-of-the-art football stadia have the facility to shield players as well as spectators from the weather outdoors. In 2003, the FA Cup final at the Millennium Stadium, Cardiff, was played under a closed roof, for the first occasion in the history of the competition. Similarly, a lack of snowfall for major skiing competitions can be countered by the production of artificial snow.

An example of how technology can assist in daring attempts was provided by Worthy[1] who described support systems for an attempt to break the world altitude record for ballooning. Two pilots were prepared to take a helium-filled balloon to a height of 39.6 km above the earth. The balloon was about 600 times bigger than the normal hot air type, needing a large volume to displace enough air to give the balloon lift once it reached the upper atmosphere's thin air. The attempt was scheduled to take 11 hours, with the pilots sitting in an open deck wearing fully pressurized space suits. The mission was prepared for the extreme low temperatures (-70°C at 20-24 km) and solar radiation. The flight platform was fitted with communication and life support equipment, within easy reach of the pilots strapped into their ergonomically designed seats. Their space suits weighed 10 kg, beneath which were thermal protective layers. The platform was rotated slowly so the pilots experienced alternating sunlight and darkness, and they were sheltered from extremes of temperature by wind deflectors and sunshields fitted to the platform. The British pilots acclimatized by undergoing altitude training in a chamber in Russia. They followed a low residue diet before the flight to reduce wastage and drank only small amounts of water through tubes inside their helmet, fed from two pouches on their suits. Notwithstanding this comprehensive attention to detail, the timing of the record attempt was dependent on favourable weather.

ACCLIMATIZATION AND HABITUATION

The sense of belonging to and fitting into the home environment is not simply one of subjective impression and general well-being. In hostile environments it reflects a physiological matching between the local inhabitants and the prevailing conditions. Suitably prepared, the sojourner may tolerate extreme conditions; even so, he or she will not achieve the physiological responses shown by the locals.

There are important physiological adjustments that take place in order to allow the individual to cope with the environment. Examples are the increase in ventilation at altitude, the bradycardia when underwater, vasodilation and sweating in the heat, vasoconstriction and raised metabolic rate in the cold. If exposure is continued, the different physiological changes are integrated so that the individual can now tolerate a sustained stay in those conditions. Applied to altitude it will mean being better able to maintain activity under the prevailing environmental stress. This process of accommodation is known as acclimatization.

In preparing for exercise in a hostile environment, the individual may train in conditions which simulate certain features of the environment to be experienced. Generally this approach entails simulation of the conditions, in an artificial environment or climate chamber. In preparing for the heat, athletes may use sweat suits, steam rooms or environmental chambers in which temperatures and humidity may be varied systematically. In preparing for altitude, they may use hypobaric rooms or normobaric hypoxic chambers. The physiological changes that result from these regimens are referred to as acclimation. The essential difference between acclimation and acclimatization is the fact that the former is artificial, the latter natural.

Individuals may benefit from undergoing simulations of hostile environments without requiring any major physiological adjustments: other than the acute responses on first exposure, they gain a subjective impression of what conditions are like in the real situation. Athletes gaining 'heat experience' in this way can plan their competition pace accordingly and be less daunted by an uncertainty of not knowing how they will feel. The sub-aqua club diver can become familiar with nitrogen narcosis in a compression chamber (see Chapter 5) and become aware of how mood and decision-making will be altered at depths underwater.[2]

Whilst sojourners acquire acclimatization to environmental conditions, they never gain the physiological characteristics that are associated with long-term dwellers. The dominance of Ethiopian and Kenyan distance runners over the last three decades has been linked with living their lives at altitude. Whether the supremacy is attributable to an evolutionary effect, to having been born at altitude (so implying that early experience can influence the body's physiology throughout life), or to the natural ability to train more intensely than sea-level dwellers, has not been fully established. At higher altitudes Peruvian highlanders display a right-ventricular hypertrophy and enhanced pulmonary diffusing capacity that do not develop in typical 'acclimatized' visitors. The local inhabitants live close to the limit of long-term habituation, and have a tradition of periodically allowing blood-letting. This practice usually coincides with when erythrocytes approach high values and haematocrit is dangerously high. Their counterparts in the Himalayas, the Sherpas, have impressed those in the mountaineering world with their capabilities to work hard in the high peaks. Clearly the successes of the majority of climbing expeditions to the highest mountain ranges on the planet have been dependent on the support work of the Sherpas.

The process of a long-term adjustment to the environment which results from living there is referred to as habituation. It combines changes attributable to evolution with the behaviour appropriate for survival. The Ama and the Eskimo are examples of habituation to cold conditions; the adjustments allow members of the former to dive in cold water and the latter to survive in permanent cold. The Eskimo uses appropriate clothing and maintains a well-insulated igloo as a home. Nevertheless, experience teaches the Eskimos to abandon sledging outdoors if feeling too cold and to run for a while to raise body temperature.[3]

There are examples also of habituation to extreme heat. The physiology of desert dwellers has been studied by Edholm and Baccharach.[4] Groups studied have included the Kalahari Bushmen, the Saharan Fulani and the Australian Aborigines. The physiological changes are only part of the capability to survive in diverse conditions. There must also be sensitive use of lifestyle and knowledge about the locations of oases when nomads are on the move. Their long loose robes allow air to circulate around the skin, keeping the body surface cool. (This strategy contrasts with the athlete competing for a short time in the heat, who can afford to expose more of the skin surface to the air to promote cooling.) Also there is a tendency amongst many to wear white – reflecting the sun's heat. When dark clothing is worn it is for cultural reasons, or because of limitations in the bleaching of materials.

ANALYZING LIFESTYLE

Seasonal influences

All regions of the Earth show marked seasonal variation, except those at, or very close to, the Equator. Seasons are caused by the elliptical orbit of the Earth around the sun and the axis of the daily rotation of the Earth being inclined at 23.5° from the vertical. This astronomical characteristic produces variation in both the duration of daylight and the angle at which the rays of the sun strike the surface of the Earth, and causes a seasonal variation in climate.

There are many different climates on Earth, with most varying to some degree with the time of year. As one moves away from the tropical, forested equatorial regions, one travels through the sub-tropical belt of hot deserts, then through a temperate region of mild winters and cool summers to reach, eventually, the polar regions of extremely cold winters and 'summers' which are still just a few degrees above 0°C. As one travels away from the equatorial regions, the climate generally becomes more seasonal, and the length of daylight within a 24-hour period deviates progressively from the constant 12 hours observed at the Equator. This deviation is most apparent close to the Earth's poles. For example, the Norwegian town of Alta (latitude 69° 58' north) experiences 24 hours of complete darkness for two months in the winter, but between the 18th of May and the 24th July, the entire sun is above the horizon for 24 hours per day. There is a large seasonal variation in climate also in temperate regions that are far from the sea (e.g. Moscow in Russia). The fact that such regions of the Earth are populated by, among others, athletes, illustrates the importance of considering the effects of seasonal variations in climate and day length.

The activity habits of populations are very much dependent on climatic conditions. The distinction between winter sports and summer sports is manifest in having separate Olympic Games for each. There is also a tradition of having seasonal sports, such as Rugby Union and cross-country in the winter, and cricket and lawn bowls in the summer. The distinction has become blurred when indoor sports facilities permit sports like tennis all the year round and 'dry-court training' for the winter sports takes place in the summer. Currently, the physical activities of individuals are no longer as tightly bound to seasonal changes as they had been for thousands of years.

There are established seasonal effects on birth rates, recreational activity, body composition, and behaviour and physical fitness. Human sexual activity tends to peak towards the end of the summer when plasma levels of circulating testosterone reach a seasonal maximum. Participation in active recreation in Scotland shows a dense peak in July and a trough in December. Seasonal changes in body composition are complex, in that an increase may reflect tendencies to increase energy intake and decrease energy output in the winter compared to summer. Yet resting metabolism is raised in winter due to secretion of thyroxine and there is a greater utilization of free fatty acids as fuel for exercise, so these mechanisms should help to release body fat in winter. Behaviour is reflected in activity patterns; non-natives living in the Arctic regions undergo a relative hibernation in winter. The same is not true for Canadian Eskimos who tend to maintain their hunter-gatherer existence in the winter months.

A pronounced seasonal effect is noted in the diurnal rhythm of melatonin secretion.[5] The hormone regulates the circadian rhythm in humans and is secreted during darkness and inhibited by outdoor light. The long hours of darkness lead to a depression (in vulnerable individuals) which is referred to as Seasonal Affective Disorder. Whereas bright light has been used as therapy for this condition, it is not known whether exercise therapy, and even a reduced secretion of melatonin, are reasonable alternatives.

Shiftwork

Like transmeridian travel, participation in shiftwork can disrupt human circadian rhythms and has deleterious effects upon training and competitive sports performance. It should be noted that crossing time-zones and working shifts are not chronobiologically identical. When multiple time-zones are crossed, a person is normally exposed to all the zeitgebers (or 'time-givers') of the new environment, whereas during rotating shiftwork that includes nightwork, any change in the phasing of a person's rhythms has occurred while being exposed to some zeitgebers still associated with a diurnal existence (e.g. the light-dark cycle). Any consideration of shiftwork is further complicated by the fact that the rhythm disturbances may not be isolated events, as in transmeridian travel, but can be frequent, occurring every time a shift may rotate.[5]

Shiftwork in some form has been practised throughout history. Baking bread and doing sentry duties of old have their current counterparts in milk deliveries and postal workers, being on permanent early morning shifts. Factory workers, taxi drivers and many others operate on rotating shifts while others may choose to stay on permanent night hours.

Nearly one-fifth of the labour force in Europe and North America is on some form of shiftwork system, mostly working irregular hours. Invariably some of these workers will be athletes. The adjustment of the circadian rhythms to nocturnal work is never complete, since the natural light-dark cycle remains unaltered in spite of changes in the zeitgeber effect of artificial light. At the top level of competitive sport, the difficulties of organizing training and competitive arrangements around a nocturnal work regimen would militate against achieving excellence. Some workers fail to adapt to permanent shiftwork and those who are susceptible suffer from adverse effects, even though they were previously healthy, including stomach ulcers and gastrointestinal symptoms. For those individuals who do cope, a forward rotating shift system, in which the sequence of hours worked becomes later on successive shifts, is preferable. The reason is that the body clock adapts more easily to a phase delay (as also happens when travelling westwards across multiple time zones) than to a phase advance.

ENVIRONMENTAL STRESSES IN COMBINATION

Environmental stresses can be considered separately in detail, as has been done in the previous chapters. This focus can help identify the physiological consequences of exposure and how athletes can prepare for features of the environment to be encountered. In reality, however, individual stresses are rarely experienced in isolation but are usually encountered in combinations.

To give some examples of common combinations: both the ambient temperature and the relative humidity decrease with increasing altitude; cold is also a corollary of deep sea-diving; the acclimatization to hot humid conditions differs in detail from acclimatization to hot dry conditions, even if the total thermal load can be compared by calculating corrected effective temperature; and noise is generally distracting but in certain circumstances can offset the soporific effect of working in the heat. Other combinations are more detrimental, such as when heat and pollution co-exist as environmental stressors during competition.

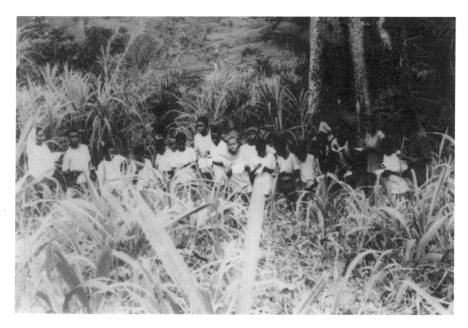

Figure 10.3 Secondary school students in Cameroon prepare for orienteering in equatorial forest

The interactions between many of the factors separately dealt with already have been the subject of investigation. An example is the study by Buguet et al.[6] who compared responses of European and African residents of the Sahel to heat: measurements were made in the dry season and responses during both the cool and hot periods were investigated. The amplitude of the circadian rhythm in rectal temperature did not vary between hot and dry periods. This finding contradicts the view that the amplitude of the rectal temperature cycle is conditioned by the ambient temperature, being greater in cold conditions (since the core temperature falls more at night) than in hot ones. No difference in rhythms was found between African and Caucasian subjects, both groups showing evidence of a similar seasonal acclimatization to heat.

The relationship between the environment, the individual and the activity is often delicately poised. The nomadic women of Southern Iran annually take their herds into the hills long distances over arid terrain to new grazing fields. The trek is long and arduous. Each year they become amenorrhoeic prior to the journey, in effect seeming to make a biological preparation for it. It appears that within the recurring menstrual cycles over the whole year, there is a sub-harmonic during which the secretion of reproductive hormones is suppressed in this nomadic group of women. This phenomenon is comparable with the secondary amenorrhoea of the endurance athlete, likely representing physiological adjustments to cope with activities rather than a damaging consequence of them.

Not all seemingly unforgiving environments prohibit sport and recreational activities. Football is undoubtedly the most popular sport worldwide and has participants in the game in some form in all continents, irrespective of climatic conditions or economic status. Some sports remain specific to local and national cultures, whilst others cross continental and environmental boundaries without great difficulty. The use of orienteering as an educational medium can be as apt in the equatorial forests as it is amongst the pine trees of Scandinavia (see Figure 10.3). 'Stick and ball' games have evolved for play on ice, grass and on contemporary synthetic surfaces. Games such as lacrosse and field hockey have their origins among North American Indians and ancient Chinese traditions respectively, and have transferred to other continents and cultures with ease.[7] However the Gaelic game of hurling which may even have predated the original form of hockey, still flourishes as a major national sport in Ireland, being hardly ever played by other ethnic groups.

CONCLUSION

The environment has been broadly investigated, embracing indoor and outdoor contexts, urban and rural contrasts, seasonal and circadian variations. The human population considered to interact with it is heterogeneous, including young or old, female or male, fit or sedentary, an elite or a novice sports participant. Whilst physiological responses to novel environments are mostly considered in terms of the typical or the average, there may be large variations between individuals in their ability to cope. Therefore, for any environmental stress, it is important to remember that there will be good and poor responders, some who will cope easily and others who will suffer greatly. The identification of those unsuitable for conditions in hostile environments is as much a challenge to the physiologist as is the identification of those that are suitable.

Training methods have been adapted to cope with environmental exigencies. Inhabitants in the cold Northern climates recognise the need to protect against the cold, and that activity can promote health rather than damage in their circumstances. The use of indoor sports facilities has been a benefit to those wishing to maintain fitness in winter-time. As yet, only a minority of natives of hot climates benefit from air-conditioned sports facilities. Facilities in the future might incorporate the creation of 'virtual reality' in which training would occur. Such options might extend to the shift-worker whose well-being could be aided by the availability of a mini-gymnasium, perhaps even at home.

Irrespective of the challenges and risks posed by environmental stress, there is an indomitable streak in humans which encourages them to overcome such adversities. The motivation to do so should not be underestimated. Nevertheless, the enthusiasm and drive to replace old boundaries should always be tempered with a consideration of the chances of success, and a detailed visualization of the things that might go wrong and the procedures that need to be in place to minimize the risk of tragedy.

References

1. Worthy T. Ergonomics gets a huge lift from flight to the edge of space. Ergonomist 2003; 397(July):1-3
2. Thomas V, Reilly T. Effects of compression on human performance and affective states. Brit J Sports Med 1974; 8:188-190
3. Shephard RJ. Alive man. Springfield: CC Thomas, 1971
4. Edholm OG, Baccharach AL. Exploration medicine. Bristol: John Wright and Sons, 1965
5. Reilly T, Atkinson G, Waterhouse J. Biological rhythms and exercise. Oxford: Oxford University Press, 1997
6. Buguet A, Gati R, Soubiron G et al. Seasonal changes in circadian rhythms of body temperatures in humans living in a dry tropical climate. Europ J Appl Physiol 1988; 250:475
7. Reilly T, Borrie A. Physiology applied to field hockey. Sports Med 1992; 14:10-26

Index

Page numbers for figures and other non-textual material are in **bold** print

A

Aborigines 45, 186
Abruzzi, Duke of 55
Acceleration forces
    angular acceleration 132
    effects 121–2
    fairgrounds 10, 121, 132
    headward acceleration 122–3, 124, **125**
    see also G-forces
Accidents 2, 6
Acclimation 25, 185
Acclimatization
    altitude 58, 61, 66, 70, 184
    characteristics of process **23**
    to cold 44
    hostile environments 185, 188
    hot conditions 22–5, 188
    pre-acclimatization strategies 23
    zero-G 136–7
Achilles tendon reflex 134
ACTH 65
Adaptation
    altitude stress 63–6
    cold conditions 44–5
    metabolic (hypoxia) 65
    ozone, effects of 155
Adenosine triphosphate 37
Adipose tissue 14, 41, 48
Adrenal cortex 65
Adrenal glands 37
Adrenaline 37, 44, 95
Adrenal medulla 124
Adrenocortical hormones 37
Age
    hearing loss 171

thermoregulatory factors 27–8
Air bubbles 84–5
Air quality 145–63
    allergens 160
    human factor 156–8
    ions 158–9
    primary pollutants 146–53
    secondary pollutants 146, 153–6
Air velocity, measurement 28
Akerstedt, T 105
Alaska, Iditarod sled-races 182
Albuquerque 66
Alcohol 24, 36
Aldosterone 22, 65
Aldrin, Buzz 117
Allen, Brian 8–9
Allergens 160
Alta (Norway) 187
Altitude stress 51–72
    acclimatization 58, 61, 66, 70, 184
    acute adaptations 63–5
    extreme altitude 55–8
    high altitudes 58–60
    illnesses **59**
    metabolic adaptations 65–6
    moderate altitudes 60–1
    non-response to training 69–70
    physiological background 52–4
    simulated altitude 67–9
    training camps 52, 61, 66–7, 184
    see also Hypoxia
Alton Towers Leisure Park 10
Ama (pearl divers) 75
Amenorrhoea, and jet lag 100
American College of Sports Medicine 29
American football 2
American Medical Research Expedition
(Everest) 57
Amphetamines 105
Anaerobic exercise 65, 66

Anal sphincter 17
Anderson, E 149
Andrenocorticoid hormones 44
Animal models 129
Annual rolling mean 151
Antarctica 40
Anthropometry 2
Antigens 160
Antigravity suits 127, 141
Antihistamines 160
Apical alveoli 125
Apocrine glands 15
Apollo 13 spacecraft 117
Aranow, W 150
Arbitrary zero 166
Arctic Circle 45
Armstrong, Neil 117
Armstrong, S 106
Arterioles 119
Asthma 147, 160
Astronauts 117, 118, 119
    diets 139
    Earth, return to 129, 137–8
    extra-vehicular activities 132
    G-forces 126
    musculo-skeletal system 135
    pre-syncope symptoms 137
    respiratory system 132
    vestibular system 133, 134
    weightlessness, effects 129, 132, 133, 134,
    135
    see also Space flights
Athens, Olympic Games (2004) 155–6
Athletes
    at altitude 70
    cold, training in 39
    drug-taking 105
    ferritin stores 64, 69–70
    fluid intake 24
    heat stress (West African) 26
    hydration status 20–1
    and Olympic Games 182
    pre-flight preparations 95
    temperature measurement 18
    time zone effects, and training 102, 104
    see also Exercise; Performance, exercise;
    Sports
Atkinson, G 150, 151
Atlanta, Olympic Games (1996) 24, 176
Atmospheric pressure 52
Atrial natriuretic peptide 65, 130
Audiometer tests 170
Auditory stimulus 165
Australia
    Aborigines 45, 186
    Barrier Reef 84

UK flights 98, 99, 100–1, 104–5, 110
Auto-cycle Union 174
Axe, J D 166
Axis of rotation 121, 122

B

Baccharach, A L 186
Baddeley, A D 81
Badminton 7
Balance, weightlessness, physiological
effects **133**
Barker, T 158, 159
Barometric pressure changes **58**
Baroreceptor reflexes 119, 124, 131
Basilar membrane (cochlea) 169
Bates, B T 9
Beamon, Bob 61, 63
Bedford, T 28
Bends 74, 85, 132
Bennett, P 79, 81, 83, 86
Benzene 146, 151
Benzodiazepines 105
Beshir, M Y 29
Binnington, J 174
'Black-out' 122, 123
Black surfaces, and heat absorption 13
Blood lactate 61–2
Body clock
    adjustment 93–4
    circadian nature 92–3
    role 94–5
    shiftwork 188
    site 92
Body fluids
    loss of (hypohydration) 19–20, 25, 26
    over-dilution (hyponatraemia) 21–2
    pooling, venous 119, **120**, 130, 141
    weightlessness, physiological effects
    129–30
Body temperature
    core *see* core body temperature
    intra-aural, measurement **17**, 18
    measurement 17–19
    nervous control of regulation **15**
    oral 18
    pre-cooling during exercise, effects 22
    rectal *see* Rectal temperature
    sublingual 18
    tympanic 17–18
    zones of responses **14**
    see also Skin temperature
Body time 109
Bogota (Columbia) 60
Bolivia, games in 60

Bone demineralization, zero-G 134–5, 137
Bone marrow 64, 70, 138
Bonington, Chris 56
Boston 149
Boxers 21
Boyle's law 74, 80, 84
BPG (bisphosphoglycerate) 64
Bradycardia 185
Brauer, M 157
Brauer, R W 83
Breath-hold diving 74, 75, 77
Bright light
    body clock adjustment 93–4
    clock-shifting **108**, 109–10
British Everest Expedition (1953) 56
British Standards Institute 79
Bronchoconstriction 158
Bronchodilators 147
Brown fat 37
Bruck, K 30
Bucher, Raimondo 77
Buenos Aires, pollution in 146
Buguet, A 189

C

Caffeine 105
Calcium 134, 139
Cameroon, orienteering **189**
Carbon dioxide
    altitude, physiological challenge caused
    by 52, 53
    breath-hold diving 77, 78
    build up of 184
    low 53
    poisoning 79, 82
    scuba diving 79
    under-water working 81
Carbon monoxide 146, 147–50
Carboxyhaemoglobin (COHb) 148, 149
Cardiff, FA Cup final (2003) 184
Cardiovascular drift 16
Cardiovascular system 124–5, 130–1
Carotid sinus 124
Case, D B 149
Cave diving 85–6
Central nervous system (CNS) 134
Centrifugal force 140
Cerebrospinal fluid 123, 169
Charry, J M 159
Chemoreceptors 53
Chibis suits 140
Chicken-leg syndrome 129
Children, thermoregulatory factors 27
Chokes 85

Cholinergic nerve fibres 15, 16
Cho Oyn (mountain) 56
Chronobiology 89, 90
Chronobiotics 106
Chronotypes 100
Cigarette smoking 148, 149
Cilia (hair cells) 169
Circadian rhythms
    air ions 158, 159
    body clock 96
    body temperature measurement 17
    chronobiology **90**
    exogenous/endogenous components 92,
    97
    light/dark cycle 8
CIS (Confederation of Independent States)
118
Clayton, J 93
Clock genes 93
Clock-shifting
    bright light **108**, 109–10
    diet/exercise 110–11
    general principles 105–6
    melatonin use 106–9
Clothing
    body heat, retention 38, 39, 40, 42, 47, 48
    dark/light 13, 186
    sweat 24–5
    water, influence on survival times in **42**
Clubbing 173
CNS (central nervous system) 134
Cochlea (inner ear) 169
COHb (carboxyhaemoglobin) 148, 149
Coin-click hearing test 169
Cold conditions, exercise in 33–49
    adaptation to 44–5
    clothing, influence on survival times in
    water 42
    coping with 38–40
    critical temperatures, biological tissues **34**
    exhaustion **44**
    hill walkers 34, 37, 38, **39**, 40
    pathologies 43–4
    performance, effect on **43**
    preparation 47
    stress, monitoring 45–7
    subjective sensation, rating scale **46**
    thermal responses, regulation **36**
    thermoregulation and 35–8
    vasodilation phenomenon **36**
    water immersion 40–3
    see also Heat, exercise in
Columbia, games in 51, 60
Competitive sport 2, 21
    see also Sports
Compression chambers **76**, 77

Computers, use in sports world 2, 3
Conduction, heat 14
Confederation of Independent States (CIS) 118
Constant-load suits 140
Convective heat exchange 13
Core body temperature
    air ions 158
    daily rhythms 90, 91
    heat exhaustion/stroke 25–6
    hypothermia 43
    maintenance 15–16
    manual dexterity 34
    rectal temperature and 17
Counter-current heat exchange 35
Cramps, heat 25
Cricket matches 7–8
'Critical incident' chain of events 6, **7**
Cromolyn sodium 147
Cryogenic gear 80
Cyclists, effect of pollution on 149–50
Cyclooxygenase inhibitors 158
Cytokine 70

D

Daily rhythms 90–5, **91**
Dalton's law 74
Damage Risk Conditions of the American
Committee of Hearing and Bioacoustics for
the Speech Frequency Range 175
Data-loggers 19
Dawson, B 24
Dawson, D 106
Deafness types 170–2
Decibels/decibel scale 166, 167
Decompression/decompression chambers
83–5, **84**
Deconditioning 131, 137
Dehydration 15, 16, 20, 21, 27, 96
Desensitisation
    ozone, effects of 155
Dexterity 34
Diaphragm 124–5
Diazepam 105
Diet 110–11, 139
Discotheques 173
Display Screen Directive 8
Distance runners 185
Diuresis 36, 65, 130
Diving
    bounce dives 82–3
    breath-hold 74, 75, 77
    cave 85–6
    competitive high 75
    fitness for 87

'hard-hat' 79
prolonged dives 75
saturation 84
scuba 75, 78, 79–80, 150
skin 75–9
Standard Diver 81
Do-it-yourself activities, effect of noise 175
Dopamine 53, 110
Drowning 41, 74, 78
Dry court training 187
Dry suits 42
Dwyer, J 86
Dyspnoea 41

E

Ear
    anatomy 167–9, 171
    buzzing in 171, 174
    deafness 170–2
    hearing tests *see* hearing tests
    protection 177–8
Eardrum 168, 169, 171
Ear muffs 177–8
Earplugs 177
Earth
    climates, variety of 186
    return from space 129, 137–8
Eccrine sweat glands 15, 16, 22
Edholm, O G 186
Edwards, B 107, 111
Electrolytes 21
Elliott, D H 79, 87
Endolymph 169
Endothelial growth factor 65
Energy-sparing concept 4
Engineering criteria, ergonomics criteria
distinguished **5**
England, P 20
Environment
    ergonomics *see* Ergonomics
    exercise and 1–11, **3**
    heat, exercise in 13–16, 24
    hostile 181–91
    standardization 7–8
Environmental chambers 25, 55, 61
Environmentalists 183
Environmental Protection Agency 151, 154
Environmental stresses, combined 188–90
Environmental temperatures
    cold conditions 34
    critical, cold conditions **34**
    hill-walkers and **39**
    monitoring, hot conditions 28–9
    see also Cold conditions, exercise in; Heat,

exercise in
Epithelial cells 153
Equator 186, 187
Equipment, protective 2, 5–6
Ergonomics 1–11
    background 1–2
    engineering criteria/ergonomics criteria
    distinguished **5**
    foundations 3–4
    health and safety 4, 5–6
    hot conditions 28
    human factors criteria 1, 4–5
    human–machine interface 8–10, **9**
    noise 172–3
    person, fitting task for 2–4
    science 1
    sports participation model **3**
    stress reduction principle 4
Erythrocytes 186
Erythropoiesis/erythropoietin 65, 67, 69, 70
Eskimos 38, 40, 79, 186
Ethane-1-hydroxy-1-diphosphonate 139
Ethiopia, distance running 185
Ethylene vinyl acetate 9–10
Eustachian tube 78, 168
Evans, Lee 61
Evaporation 14–15, 16
Everest *see* Mount Everest, climbing
Exercise
    anaerobic 65, 66
    body temperature, effects of pre-cooling
    during 22
    clock-shifting 110–11
    in cold *see* cold conditions, exercise in
    and environment 1–11, **3**
    in heat *see* heat, exercise in
    hyperbaric 86
    and music 176
    performance *see* Performance, exercise
    warming up prior to 19, 39
    see also Athletes; Sports
Exhaustion
    cold conditions, exercise in **44**
    heat 22, 25, **26**
    hypothermia 43
    pollution, effect 149, 150
    travel 95–111

F

Face-masks 157
FA Cup final (2003), Cardiff 184
Fairgrounds 10, 121, 132
Fanger, P O 29
Fatigue *see* Exhaustion; Travel stress

Feeding hypothesis 110–11
Ferretti, G 77
Ficca, G 105
Fins, swim 86
First stage alert, ozone pollution 154
Fleming, N C 81
Fletcher, H 167
Flights, long-distance
    before travel 95, 103
    during travel 95–6, 103–4
    following travel 96, 104–11
    jet lag *see* Jet lag
    time zones *see* Time zones
Folinsbee, L J 148, 149, 155
Four Inns walking disaster 38
Frequencies, noise 166, 172
Frostbite 40, 44
Fulani, Saharan 186

G

Gagarin, Yuri 117
Galloway, S D R 34
Gauer-Henry reflex 130
Gender, thermoregulatory factors 27–8
Georghiou, P E 153
G-forces
    cardiovascular system 124–5
    countermeasures 126–7
    decreased 121
    fairgrounds 10, 121, 132
    increased 122–7, **123**
    respiratory system 124–5
    study methods 122
    tolerance to 126
    vision/consciousness, effect on 122–4, **123**
    see also Acceleration forces
Gill, R M F 150
Glaisher, J 55
Glass-wool ear plugs 177
Gliding 52, 60
Global warming 184
GLUT-1 transporter 65–6
Glutamate 94
Goggles 78, 127
Golden, F 41
Gossamor machines 8–9
Grandjean, E 4
Grant-White 152
Gravity, effects 119–22, **120**, 128
    artificial 140
'Grey-out' 122
Grievink, L 158
Grip strength, daily rhythms **91**
Grobler, S R 152

Gulf of Mexico 55

H

Habeler, Peter 56
Habituation 186
Hackney 155
Haematocrit 65, 66, 67, 186
Haemoglobin 54, 64–5, 66, 67, 147
Hamster experiments 111
Hang-gliding 52, 60
Hawkins, L H 158, 159
Hay fever 160
Hazardous sports 2
Head injuries 170
Headward acceleration, effect 122–3, 124, **125**
Health and Safety at Work Act 1974 5, 174
Health and safety, ergonomics 4, 5–6
Hearing tests
    clinical 170
    simple 169–70
Heart rate, weightlessness, physiological effects **131**
Heat, exercise in 13–31
    acclimatization 22–5, 188
    age/gender 27–8
    body temperature see body temperature
    disorders, characteristics **26**
    environment 13–16
    exchange mechanisms **14**
    habituation 186
    injury 25–6
    performance, effects on 19–22
    thermoregulation 16
    vulnerable individuals **26**
    see also Cold conditions, exercise in
Heat exhaustion 22, 25, **26**
Heat gain centre 35
Heat stroke 25–6
Heat syncope **26**
Helium 55, 81, 82, 86
Helmets 78, 79, 178
Hendriksen, I J M 68
Henry's law 74
Hertz (Hz) 166
Hessemer, V 22
HIF-1 (hypoxia-inducible factor 1) 65
High altitude deterioration 58, **59**
High pressure neurological syndrome (HPNS) 82–3
Hillary, Edmund 56
Hill-walkers, and cold conditions 34, 37, 38, **39**, 40
Himalayas 52, 55, 56
Hockey 190

Holmer, I 46–7
Horvath, S M 149, 155
Hostile environments 181–91
    acclimatization 185
    combined stresses 188–90
    habituation 186
    lifestyle 186–8
    nature, balance with 183–4
    protective equipment 5
    seasonal factors 186–7
    shiftwork 187–8
Hot-air ballooning 52, 55, 184
H.p.G (pressure difference) 126, 128, 129
HPNS (high pressure neurological syndrome) 82–3
Human Ethics Committee 5
Human factors
    air quality 156–8
    ergonomics 1, 4–5
Human–machine interface 8–10, **9**
Hydrocarbons 146, 151, 153
Hydrogen 55
Hydroxyproline 134
Hygrometer 28
Hyperbaric exercise 86
Hyperthermia (overheating) 13, 25, 27
Hyperventilation 41, 53, 58, 64, 78
Hypobaric huts 52, 185
Hypocapnia (low carbon dioxide) 53
Hypoglycaemia 37
Hypohydration (loss of body fluid) 19–20, 25, 26
Hyponatraemia (over-dilution of body fluids) 21–2
Hypothalamus 16, 35
Hypothermia
    altitude training 70
    cave diving 85
    cold conditions, exercise in **36**, 38, 40, 41, 43, 47
    immersion in water, prolonged 74
Hypoxaemia 125
Hypoxia
    adjustments on exposure to 53
    erythropoiesis 67
    extreme altitudes 55
    metabolic adaptations 65
    performance affected by 61
    symptoms 52, **59**
    see also Altitude stress
Hypoxia-inducible factor 1 (HIF-1) 65
Hypoxic exercise room, normobaric 52, 68, **69**, 185
Hypoxic huts/chambers 25, 55, 61, 67–8

I

Iceland, waterfalls **182**
Ice-skating 151
Iditarod sled-races, Alaska 182
Immunoglobulin E (IgE) 160
Inbar, O 158, 159
Incus (anvil, middle ear) 168
Indians, Central America 79
Ingjer, F 67
Injuries, heat, exercise in 25–6
Inner ear 168–9, 171
    damage 170
Insulation, clothing 38, 39, 40, 42, 47, 48
International Association of Free Divers 77
International Civil Aviation Organisation,
Standard Atmosphere 57
International Olympic Committee 105
International Organisation for
Standardisation (ISO) 7
Intra-aural temperature, measurement **17**, 18
Intracellular fluid 169
Ions 158–9
Iran, nomadic women of 189
Iron stores 64, 69–70
Ischaemia 125
Ishikawa, Tomiyasu 56
ISO (International Organisation for
Standardisation) 7
Isometric knee extension, daily rhythms **91**

J

Japan, pearl diving 75
Jet lag 89, 96–111
    advice 103–11
    alertness, promoting 105
    checklist **111**
    clock-shifting *see* clock-shifting
    duration, estimates **112**
    general lifestyle 104–5
    individual differences in experience
    99–101
    mean, measured on Visual Analogue
    Scale (VAS) **106**
    sleep and 101–2, 105
    subjective assessments 98–9
    symptoms 97–8, **99**
Jockeys 21
Johnson, Michael 176

K

K2 (mountain) 56
Kalahari Bushmen 45, 186
Kangchenjunga (mountain) 56
Karakorum Mountains 55
Karnicar, Davo 56
Keatinge, W R 43
Kenya, distance running 185
Kidney function 135
Kinaesthesia 132
Kinoshita, H 9
Kipa, Ming 56
Knee extension, daily rhythms **91**
Korea, pearl diving 75
Kyoto Agreement 184

L

Lacrosse 190
Lactate threshold 149
Lactic acid 21, 53, 64
La Paz (Bolivia) 60
Larks 100
LBNP (lower body negative pressure) 139
Lead 151–2
Lee, D H K 28, 29
Lee, K 157
Leg strength, change in local timing **102**
Lhotse (mountain) 56
Light
    artificial 8
    bright *see* Bright light
    indoor 7, 8
    sports performance 7–8
    as zeitgeber 93
Light boxes 109
Long jump 61, 63
Los Angeles Basin 146, 155, 156
Los Angeles Olympic Games (1984) 154
Lower body negative pressure (LBNP) 139
Lunar day (24.8 h) 90
Lung function 147, **154**
Lung rupture 75
Lungs, space flight, effects 125, 132

M

McCafferty, W B 157
McCombe, A W 174
Mackay, D E 79
McMurray, R G 86
Makalu (mountain) 56

Malleus (hammer, middle ear) 168
Marathon de Sable, Sahara desert 182
Marathons 22
Mars 127
Maughan, R J 34
Mean body temperature (MBT) 18
Medulla 53
Meeuwsen, T 68
Melatonin 8, 93, 94, 187
    clock-shifting 106–9
Menstrual cycle disorders, and jet lag 100
Messner, Reinhold 56
Mestre, Audrey 77
Metabolism/metabolic rate 37, 158, 159, 187
Mexico City Olympics 51, 60, 63
Microevents 101
Microgravity see Zero-G
Microsleep 101, 112
Middle ear 168, 169, 171
Miles, S 79
Minute ventilation (VE) 45, 148, 157
Mir (space station) 118, 129
Modafinil 105
Mosso, Angelo 55
Motor cycling/racing, effect of noise 174–5
Motor vehicle pollution 147, 150
Motorways 149
Mountaineering 55, 60
Mountain sickness 52
    acute 53, **59**, 60, 65, 67, 70, 150
    chronic **59**
Mount Everest, climbing 51, 56, **57**, 183
Mount Fako, West Africa 60
Moyel, Jacques 75
mRNA 93
Munson, W A 167
Muscle fatigue curve 41
Musculo-skeletal system
    weightlessness, physiological effects 121,
    134–5
Music 173–4, 176
Myhre, K 67

N

Napping 96, 112
Narcolepsy 105
National Institute of Occupational Safety
and Health (US) 29
Natural fibre 38
Nerve deafness 170
Neuroendocrine system 37
Neuropeptides 60
New York 149
Nicholson, J P 149

Niggles 85
Nitrogen 80
Nitrogen dioxide 153
Nitrogen monoxide 153
Nitrogen narcosis 81, 185
Nitrogen oxides 146, 150–1
Nitrox 82
Noise 165–79
    control 176–8
        at source 176–7
    deafness 170–2
    ear, anatomy 167–9, 171
    ear protection 177–8
    ergonomics 172–3
    hearing tests 169–70
    high-pitched 172–3
    isolation of 177
    low-pitched 173
    physics 166–7
Noise Advisory Council 175
Noradrenaline 35, 110
Norgay, Tensing 56
Normobaric hypoxic rooms 52, 68, **69**, 185
Norton, I M 56

O

Octopush 75, 81
Oedema, pulmonary/cerebral 59, 65, 78, 125
Olympic Games 182, 187
    1968 (Mexico City) 51, 60, 63
    1984 (Los Angeles) 154
    1996 (Atlanta) 24, 176
    2004 (Athens) 155–6
1-G 119, 121
Open circuit breathing apparatus, scuba
    diving 79–80, 82
Opto-electronic devices 18
Opto-kinetic reflexes 132, 133, 137, 138
Organ of Corti 169
Orienteering 190
Orthostatic hypotension (dizziness) 119
Oschewski, H 22
Osmolality 20–1, 24
Ossicles 169, 171
Otoliths 121, 132, 133, 134
Outer ear 168
Owls 100
Oxidative phosphorylation 134
Oxygen
    alveolar–arterial difference **62**
    carboxyhaemoglobin, increasing, effect
    on uptake **148**
    dissociation curve of haemoglobin 54
    and ozone 153

partial pressure (PO$_2$) 52, **53**, **58**, 64, 77, 78
    saturation 54, 64
    scuba diving 80
    supplementary, use 5–6
    toxicity 81–2
Oxyhaemoglobin saturation **58**
Oxyhelium 81, 83
Ozone 146, 153–6, **154**

P

P4SR (4-hour sweat rate) 28
Pan American Games, Mexico (1955) 60
PAN (peroxyacetyl nitrate) 146, 156
Parachuting 52, 60
'Paradise' 181
Parathyroid hormone 135, 138
Parsons, K C 7
Passel, C F 45
Pellizeri, Umberto 75, 77
Pemoline 105
Penguin suits 140
Performance, exercise
    air ions, effect 158
    altitude, effects 61–3
    COHb levels, effect 149
    cold conditions, effects **43**
    fluid loss, effect on 20
    heat, effects 19–22
    matching light characteristics 7–8
    music, influence of 176
    sleep loss, effects 101–2, 112
    see also Athletes; Exercise; Sports
Perilymph 169
Peroxyacetyl nitrate (PAN) 146, 156
Persian Gulf, pearl divers in 78
Petrol, unleaded 151
Phase response curve (PRC) 108
Phons/phon scale 167
Phosphofructokinase 66
Pilot fatigue 101
Pineal gland 8, 93
Pinna (external ear) 168
Pituitary gland 21, 37, 65
PM-10s 146, 153
Pollution
    energy utilization 145
    human characteristics 156–7
    noise 165
        see also Noise
    preventive measures 157–8
    primary pollutants 146–53
    secondary pollutants 146, 153–6
Polynesian waters, pearl diving in 78
Polypropylene 39

Positive-pressure breathing 126
Posture, weightlessness, physiological effects
    133
Power napping 96, 112
PRC (phase response curve) 108
Prefabricated ear plugs 177
Presbyacousis 171
Pre-syncope symptoms 137
Probes, core temperature measurement 17
Protective equipment 2, 5–6
Pugh, L G C E 38

R

Race-track 174
Raphé nucleus 110
Raven, P B 149, 155
Recreational activities, noise effects 173–6
Rectal temperature 17, 38–9, **92**, 158, 159
Red blood cells 64, 66, 67, 135
Redfern, P 106
Reilly, T 10, 25, 90, 158, 159
Renal calculi 135
Renin 65
Renin-angiotensin-aldosterone axis 130
Rescue crews 48
Respiratory alkalosis 41, 53, 54, 59
Respiratory system 74, 121, 124–5, 132
    see also Lung function; Lung rupture;
    Lungs
Reticulocytes 138
Retinohypothalamic tract 94
Rodent experiments 111
Ross and Prather 55
Rotation, axis of 121, 122
'Round the World' races 184
Rugby Union 51
Runners 149, 185

S

SAD (Seasonal Affective Disorder) 187
Safety factors, ergonomics 4, 5–6
Sahara desert, Marathon de Sable 182
Saltin, B 65, 66
Salyut I spacecraft 117, 129
Samel, A 101
Samet, J 157
Saunas 25
Schematic work station analysis map **6**
SCN (suprachiasmatic nuclei) 92, 93, 94
Scotland, pollution in 146
Scuba diving 75, 78, 79–80, 150
Seasonal Affective Disorder (SAD) 187

Second stage alert, ozone pollution 154
Semicircular canals 121–2, 134
Serotonin 158
Shannon, K 166
Sherpas 186
Shiftwork 187–8
Shivering 37, 43
Shoes, sports 9–10
Shooting 152, 174
Shuttle flights **131**
Siberia 40
Sine waves 166
Sinuses, blocked 74
Siple, P A 45
Skiers 34, 51, 60, 67, 183
Skin diving 75–9
Skin temperature 33–4, 35
Skull fractures 170
Skylab spacecraft 117, 118, 129, **131**
Sleep (jet lag) 101–2, 105
Smoking 148, 149
Snorkels 78, 79
Snow blindness 70
Snowmobiling, effect of noise 175
Soccer 8, **22**, 24, 51
Solar day (24-h) 90, 93
Sommervell, P 56
Sound waves 166, 169, 171
South Africa
    games in 51, 60
    lead concentrations 152
    UK, flights from 95
Soviet Union 118
Sovijarvi, A R A 158, 159
Soyuz spacecraft 118, 129
Space Age 117
Space flights 117–43
    acceleration forces see Acceleration forces
    Earth, return to 129, 137–8
    G-forces see G-forces
    gravity, effects 119–22, 120
    human-machine interface 8–9
    recovery times following 138
    tourist flights 118
    weightlessness see Weightlessness,
    physiological effects
    see also Astronauts
Spacelab 129
Space suits 140, 184
Space tourism **118**, 119
Speech audiometry 170
Spitzer, R 98, 107
Sports
    competitive 2, 21
    hazardous 2
    noise effects 173–6

underwater see Underwater sports
    see also Athletes; Exercise; Performance,
    exercise
Sports drinks 21
Sports injuries 35
Sports participation, ergonomics model **3**
Sprinters 22
Sputnik I 117
Squirrel data-logger 19
Staggers 85
Stapedius muscles 169
Stapes (stirrup, middle ear) 168
Starling's law 124
Sterilization fluid 17
Stevenson 158, 159
Stevenson screen 28
'Stick and ball' games 190
Stromme, S B 152
Subcutaneous adipose tissue 14, 41, 48
Sulphur dioxide/sulphur trioxide 146–7
Summer sports 187
Sunburn 23, 181
Suprachiasmatic nuclei (SCN) 92, 93, 94
Sweat
    contents 21
    heat acclimatization 22, 24
    loss of 19–20
    P4SR (4-hour sweat rate) 28
Sweat clothing 24–5, 185
Sweat glands 15, 16, 22
Swimmers 18, 41–3, 48, 150
Swimming pools
    indoor 75, 175
    noise, effect of 175
    temperature 40–1

T

Tabei, Junko 56
Tectorial membrane (cochlea) 169
Temazepam 104, 105
Temperature see Body temperature;
    Environmental temperatures
Temperature equivalents 46
Temporary threshold shifts (TTS) 175
Tensor tympani 169
Terrados, N 68
Thermal responses, regulation **36**
Thermogenesis 37
Thermoregulation 16, 35–8, 75, 158–9
Thirst 20, 23
Thoracic squeeze 78
Thyroid gland 37
Thyroxine 44
Time zones (long-distance flights)

brief stays 103
little change in 95–6
longer stays 103–11
multiple, crossing 188
rapid transitions 96–111, **97**, **98**
shiftwork compared 187–8
slow transition 111–13
UK/Australia 98, 99, 100–1, 105, 110
UK/South Africa 95
Tindall, N 150
Tipton, M J 41
Tissandier, O 55
Tourism, space **118**, 119
Towse, E J 81
Training camps
altitude 52, 61, 66–7, 184
warm-weather 24, 25
Transmural pressure 119, 129
Travel stress 89–115
daily rhythms 90–5, **91**
fatigue 89, 95–111
checklist **97**
jet lag *see* jet lag
time zones *see* time zones (long-distance flights)
Trekkers 183
Trench-foot 40
Triathlons 22
Trimix 83
Tsheri, Temba 56
TTS (temporary threshold shifts) 175
Turkish baths 25
Tympanic body temperature 17–18
Tympanic membrane (eardrum) 168, 169, 171

U

Ultrasound 166
Unconsciousness 122, 124
Undergarments 39
Underwater sports 73–88
bradycardia 185
cave diving 85–6
decompression 83–5, **84**
density of gas 80–1
diving, fitness for 87
hyperbaric exercise 86
pressure/volume changes 80
scuba diving 75, 79–80
skin diving 75–9
stress 74–5
working underwater, consequences 80–3
see also Water immersion
Union of Soviet Socialist Republics (USSR) 118
United Kingdom

Australia, flights to 98, 99, 100–1, 105, 110
lead levels 152
ozone 153
South Africa, flights to 95
United States
American College of Sports Medicine 29
American football 2
National Institute of Occupational Safety and Health 29
pollution 146, 149
ozone 153, 155
space travel 117, 118
Urea 21
Urine 18, 23, 24
osmolality 20–1, 24
USSR (Union of Soviet Socialist Republics) 118

V

Valsalva manoeuvre 126
Van Rensburg, J P 152
Vasoconstriction
altitude stress 53
cold, adaptation to 35, 37, 44–5, 185
water immersion 41
Vasodilation
altitude stress 53
cold 33, 35, **36**, 45
heat 16, 185
VDUs (visual display units) 8
Veins 119–20
VE (minute ventilation) 45, 148, 157
Venous pooling 119, **120**, 130, 141
Ventilation/perfusion ratio 125
Ventricular fibrillation 43
Vestibular system 122, 132–4, 137, 138
Vibrations 168
Virtual reality environments 2, 3, 190
Vision 7, 122–4, **123**
Visual Analogue Scale (VAS) **106**
Visual display units (VDUs) 8
Vitamin C 157–8
Vitamin D 135, 138, 139
Vitamin E 157
Voice and whisper hearing test 169

W

Waldman, M 149, 150
Warming up 19, 39
Watch-tick hearing test 169
Waterhouse, J M 122
Water immersion

clothing, influence on survival times **42**
cold conditions, exercise in 40–3
diuresis 130
nausea and 133
prolonged 74
rationale for 128
see also Swimmers; Swimming pools;
Underwater sports
WBGT (wet bulb, globe temperature) Index
24, 28–9
Weightlessness, physiological effects 127–41
balance **133**
body fluids 129–30
cardiovascular system 130–1
Earth, return to 129, 137–8
mean heart rate measurements **131**
musculo-skeletal system 134–5
posture **133**
respiratory system 132
study methods 128–9
vestibular system 132–4
zero-G *see* zero-G
Weight loss 21
West Africa, heat stress 26
Wet suits 42, 74–5
White blood cells 135
Windbreakers 24
Wind chill formula, heat loss 45, **46**
Wind noise 174
Winter sports 33, 187
Workplace design, classical model 5, **6**

Work-rate, self-selected, daily rhythms **91**
World Conference on Underwater Activities 77
World Cup soccer tournaments 24, 51
World Health Organisation 151
Worthy, T 184
Wrestlers 21

Y

Yosemite Valley **183**

Z

Zeitgebers (time-givers) 93, 94, 107, 188
Zenith (French balloon) 55
Zero-G environment
acclimatization 136–7
bone demineralization 134–5
cardiovascular 'deconditioning' 131
changes during **136**
countermeasures 139–41, **140**
description 121
minor operations 136
respiratory system 132
vestibular system 133, 134
see also Weightlessness, physiological
effects
Zolpiden 104